# ESSENTIALS IN CYTOPATHOLOGY

*Dorothy L. Rosenthal, MD, FIAC, Series Editor*

**Editorial Board**

*Syed Z. Ali, MD*
*Douglas P. Clark, MD*
*Yener S. Erozan, MD*

More information about this series at
http://www.springer.com/series/6996

Rosemary H. Tambouret
David C. Wilbur

# Glandular Lesions
# of the Uterine Cervix

## Cytopathology
## with Histologic Correlates

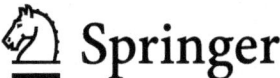 Springer

Rosemary H. Tambouret, MD
Department of Pathology
Massachusetts General Hospital
Boston, MA, USA

David C. Wilbur, MD
Department of Pathology
Massachusetts General Hospital
Boston, MA, USA

ISSN 1574-9053            ISSN 1574-9061 (electronic)
ISBN 978-1-4939-1988-8    ISBN 978-1-4939-1989-5 (eBook)
DOI 10.1007/978-1-4939-1989-5
Springer New York Heidelberg Dordrecht London

Library of Congress Control Number: 2014949780

Printed on acid-free paper

Springer is part of Springer Science+Business Media (www.springer.com)

# Foreword

I am delighted to contribute the foreword to this book written by two colleagues who are not only good friends but also outstanding diagnostic pathologists who have assisted me greatly over the years. I also consider it highly appropriate that a book on cytopathology of the uterine cervix be coauthored by two members of the cytopathology laboratories of the Massachusetts General Hospital, Harvard Medical School, given the very significant role the unit played in the acceptance of cytopathology as a discipline in the United States. Some readers may not know that when cytopathology was entering the field of anatomic pathology as a subdiscipline, it received much initial opposition from many traditional diagnostic pathologists, including the then chief of pathology of the Massachusetts General Hospital (MGH), Dr. Tracy Mallory. That they might have some reservations about the "new kid on the block" was perhaps not surprising, and we should not cast any aspersions on that distinguished pathologist or others who felt as he did. Nonetheless, it has been to the great benefit of medicine, and more importantly the populace at large, that others felt differently, including the pioneering gynecologic oncologist Dr. Joe V. Meigs. As Dr. Wilbur has recounted elsewhere, he was approached by an MGH internist, Dr. Maurice Fremont-Smith, after the latter visited the laboratory of Dr. Papanicolaou in New York, and he was intrigued by what he saw. Dr. Meigs was of an innovative disposition, saw the potential benefit of the technique quicker than many, and recruited the pioneering cyto-technologist Ruth M. Graham to help implement cytopathology in practice in Boston. The first cytology laboratory at this hospital was accordingly established in the gynecology service of the MGH (then and now known as the Vincent Memorial Hospital) in 1942 and was the first such cytology laboratory established in this country after that of Dr. Papanicolaou himself. The work of the early investigators at the MGH was noted by the American Medical Association when, in 1944, they honored them with a certificate of merit because of their work (the honor being shared with Cornell Medical Center). The elegant diploma still is displayed in the cytology laboratories of this institution. Further note might be made of the fact that Ruth Graham and her staff published the first textbook of cytology in 1950. As will be evident from these remarks, Dr. Tambouret and Dr. Wilbur are part of a great tradition, and I can certainly, based on my own personal knowledge of their expertise, simply note that they are upholding this noble tradition in a most outstanding manner on a daily basis and by their efforts both nationally and internationally. Cytology only transitioned to pathology at this institution in the mid-1950s, and has resided there from that time, Dr. Wilbur serving as director of the unit for a number of years beginning in 2001 until, voluntarily, he passed on the torch. He remains fully active in the unit, signing out on a regular basis, as does Dr. Tambouret, and both are mainstays of the general gynecologic pathology diagnostic histopathology service.

That this text covers glandular lesions of the uterine cervix is itself noteworthy, inasmuch as the early pioneers focused largely on squamous lesions. It is only since the mid- to late 1970s that progressively greater attention has been focused on the numerous challenges provided by endocervical glandular lesions in both cytopathology and histopathology. Although of course getting coverage in various texts and other sources on occasion, glandular lesions get overwhelmed from the coverage viewpoint by the more common squamous abnormalities, and it is timely to see a work focused only on the endocervical cell. In my own practice, I see countless problematic endocervical glandular proliferations, many of which Dr. Tambouret and Dr. Wilbur assist me with, and it is not unusual for them, quite appropriately, to me wish to correlate biopsy findings with those in cytologic preparations. Considering the two can be of great benefit in arriving at the correct diagnosis. The initial evaluation of endocervical abnormalities of most patients does begin with cytologic material, and it is the first point in the chain that we all hope leads to good clinical care. Accordingly, it is obviously crucial that such specimens are appropriately evaluated so that significant lesions are not delayed in further evaluation, and from a contrary perspective, lesions of benign nature do not lead to mismanagement and undue patient anxiety. The practice of cytopathology is a visual discipline, albeit impacted of course by the eye of experience and some awareness of the clinical background including the patient age, among other things. Much as words may help in elaboration of potential pitfalls, the proverbial "picture speaks a thousand words," and accordingly, this work is liberally presented with high-quality illustrations. All who practice the discipline of cytopathology will, I am sure, find this a most instructive volume to have available, given the knowledge and experience of the writers. I am delighted to have the opportunity to make these remarks concerning this fine work.

Boston, MA, USA                    Robert H. Young
Boston, MA, USA                    Robert E. Scully

# Reference

1. Wilbur DC. Cytopathology. In: Louis DN, Young RH, editors. Keen minds to explore the dark continents of disease: a history of the pathology services at the Massachusetts General Hospital. Beverly: Memoirs Unlimited; 2011.

# Preface

The evaluation of glandular lesions in cervical cytology specimens can be vexing, even to the most experienced cytologist. The mere identification that a glandular lesion is present can be subtle during the screening process, and once a potential abnormality is detected, accurate classification can be even more challenging. Compared to the more prevalent squamous lesions, glandular lesions in cervical cytology specimens were not well recognized or fully classified until late. Endocervical adenocarcinoma in situ (AIS) was not fully described in the histopathology literature until 1953 [1], and it was not codified as a discrete cytologic entity until the second edition of the Bethesda Manual (TBS2) in 2001 [2]. Prior to that AIS was grouped under the descriptor of "atypical glandular cells of undetermined significance, favor neoplasia." In the 1990s, a number of detailed publications that appeared defined the morphologic characteristics of AIS and showed that when applied correctly, these criteria were actually predictive when histologic specimens were obtained [3–5]. Extensive study of glandular lesions followed upon the publication of TBS2 such that a variety of conditions affecting glandular cells of the gynecologic tract became better recognized and the morphologic criteria for each became better defined.

It is fair to say that there has been an increased awareness that, although the test is not perfect, glandular lesions can indeed be reliably identified in cervical cytology specimens. As with any newly emerging discipline, the ability to detect glandular lesions has had other effects. Patients now expect that, just like squamous neoplasia, glandular neoplasia can be perfectly identified when present. Many lawsuits alleging malpractice have involved this very subject. The unfortunate truth is that the Pap test is not as sensitive for endocervical as it is for squamous neoplasias. The anatomy of endocervical cell location and the plethora of reactive mimics make accurate detection difficult from both sampling and interpretation viewpoints, respectively. That being said, there is always room for improvement and that is the idea behind the present monograph.

At the Massachusetts General Hospital, we are fortunate to have access to the material from very active gynecologic oncology, colposcopy, and general screening services. In addition, there are a large number of outside consultation cases that are received for review by our subspecialty experts in gynecologic practice, both clinical and pathologic. In the writing of the text and collection of the illustrations, we have attempted to identify the key issues in the cytology of glandular lesions, to present the important demography and clinical features associated with them, and finally to describe and to illustrate the pertinent morphology of these lesions.

The monograph begins with a background discussion and illustration of the normal histology and cytology associated with glandular epithelia in the gynecologic tract. It then describes the prototypical endocervical and endometrial neoplasia spectrums. In addition, illustrations of malignant mimickers, namely metastatic adenocarcinomas, which can have appearances very similar to primary lesions will be presented, with the discussion focusing on the features that should help the observer to make a correct final interpretation. The latter morphologic chapters focus on the many mimickers of glandular neoplasia. Entities such as the large number of metaplastic processes, reactive endocervical cells caused by irritants such as polyps, intrauterine devices, prior biopsies, infectious disease, and many more will be detailed. These benign entities are common and can actually be the underlying cause of many cases of interpretations of "atypical glandular cells (AGC)." It has been a "rule of thumb" for many years that the majority of cases of AGC will turn out to be either benign/reactive or unusual presentations of squamous intraepithelial lesions, with only a small minority actually representing true glandular neoplasias. Hence recognition and correct classification of these presentations as benign can lead to significant improvements in cervical cytology specificity and can help to avoid costly and stressful follow-up clinical investigations. Therefore accuracy in both directions, detection and false negativity, as well as classification and false positivity, are addressed by this monograph.

Aids to interpretation have become very important in histopathologic applications. When applied to cytologic preparations, the use of immunohistochemistry for markers associated with high risk HPV-associated neoplastic transformation and with types of differentiation has greatly aided again, both detection and classification. The principles behind their use and illustrations to aid in proper interpretation are presented in order to bring the reader up to speed with this newly emerging functionality.

Finally, the management of glandular lesions may seem like the clinicians' domain. But it is extremely important for laboratory professionals to be aware of the published guidelines. These lesions are rare in the general screening population and the cytologist, because of their diagnostic role, may be in the best position to advise and guide the clinician trying to determine the best course of action. Therefore the newest management algorithms are presented to assist the cytologist in this important advisory role. In addition, appropriate quality assurance practices, such as prevalence monitoring, cytology–histology correlation, and HPV testing use are included as these will be important to the laboratorian.

We certainly hope that this monograph meets the needs of the cytology community and that the format and content is displayed in a manner that allows for easy access, adaptability to clinical situations, and ease of information transfer. It has been our pleasure to "put down on paper" these subjects that we have studies and struggled over for the better parts of our careers. We hope that the knowledge and experience that we have gained will be useful to the reader.

Boston, MA                    Rosemary H. Tambouret
2014                                David C. Wilbur

# References

1. Friedell GH, McKay DG. Adenocarcinoma in situ of the endocervix. Cancer. 1953;6(5):887–97.
2. Solomon D, Davey D, et al. The Bethesda System 2001: terminology for reporting the results of cervical cytology. JAMA. 2002;287:2114–9.
3. Ayer B, Pacey F, et al. The cytologic diagnosis of adenocarcinoma in situ of the cervix uteri and related lesions. I. Adenocarcinoma in situ. Acta Cytol. 1987;31(4):397–411.
4. Wilbur DC, Dubeshter B, et al. Use of thin-layer preparation for gynecologic smears with emphasis on the cytomorphology of high-grade intrapepithelial lesions and carcinomas. Diagn Cytopathol. 1996;14(3):201–11.
5. Johnson JE, Rahemtulla A. Endocervical glandular neoplasia and its mimics in Thinprep Pap tests. A descriptive study. Acta Cytol. 1999;43:369–75.

# Contents

# Chapter 1
## Introduction to Endocervical Glandular Lesions

Correct cytological interpretation of glandular lesions of the cervix has challenged cytologists for years. Cervical cytology or the Pap test was initially intended to screen for squamous carcinoma and precursor squamous lesions but with time it became evident that endocervical glandular lesions were recognizable as well. The development of cytologic criteria for the recognition of endocervical lesions lagged behind that of squamous lesions, probably in part because endocervical adenocarcinoma is less common than squamous carcinoma but also because the histologic criteria were defined at a later date. For example, in North America cytologic criteria for endocervical adenocarcinoma in situ (AIS) were only sufficiently delineated, found to be reproducible, and therefore accepted by the cytology community as late as 2004, when they were first included in the second edition of the Bethesda System manual [1, 2]. Lesser degrees of glandular dysplasia or precursor glandular lesions on cervical cytology have yet to be precisely defined either cytologically or histologically. Certainly, the early cytologic emphasis was on the more common squamous lesions; however, additional factors delayed progress with glandular neoplasia. Using early sampling devices, such as fiber swabs, far less cellular material was available for analysis from the upper portions of the endocervical canal. Therefore less cellular material from these areas

R.H. Tambouret and D.C. Wilbur, *Glandular Lesions of the Uterine Cervix*, Essentials in Cytopathology 19, DOI 10.1007/978-1-4939-1989-5_1, © Springer Science+Business Media New York 2015

led to lower sensitivities for these analyses, and less recognition and study of even benign and reactive processes were exhibited by the epithelium of the endocervical canal. This undoubtedly led to lower levels of interest, and hence less progress. The literature on glandular lesions blossomed with the advent of better sampling devices such as brooms and brushes in the late 1980s and 1990s. To some degree this increased attention became absolutely necessary as the cytologist needed to deal with the large volumes of endocervical canal-derived material and its many presentations as will be detailed in this monograph.

## Prevalence

Over the last half century or more, adenocarcinoma has made up an increasing proportion of invasive cervical cancers. A study of cervical carcinoma from 1936 to 1967 at the hospital of the University of Pennsylvania found 6.1 % of cases were adenocarcinoma [3]. In several more recent studies of cervical cancer, the rate of adenocarcinoma ranged from 20 to 25 % [4, 5].

Studies of the data collected by the National Cancer Institute's Surveillance, Epidemiology, and End Results (SEER) Program in the United States on cervical cancer incidence from 1973 to as recently as 2008 have shown that the incidence of cervical adenocarcinoma is on the rise but the rise is dwarfed by the overall decline in incidence of invasive cervical cancer due to the decreased incidence of squamous cell carcinoma [6–9]. One study analyzing the data from 1973 to 1996 found that the age-adjusted incidence rates of squamous cell carcinoma declined by 41.9 % while the age-adjusted incidence rate of adenocarcinoma increased by 29.1 % and that the proportion of adenocarcinoma relative to squamous cell carcinoma increased by 95.2 % [6]. Analysis of SEER data for years 1973–1989 showed a 14.0 % incidence of adenocarcinoma as compared to 24.2 % for the years 1990–2008 resulting in a 1.95 times higher odds ratio of a newly diagnosed cervical cancer being adenocarcinoma during the later period as compared to the earlier period (Table 1.1) [7].

TABLE 1.1 Incidence of cervical cancer over 35 years in the United States using the National Cancer Institute's Surveillance, Epidemiology, and End Results (SEER) Program [7]

| | 1973–1989 | | 1990–2008 | | Change per 100,000 women | |
|---|---|---|---|---|---|---|
| | N (%) | 95 % CI | N (%) | 95 % CI | EAPC | 95 % CI |
| Total | 19,907 (100.0) | – | 20,456 (100.0) | – | −2.3 | −2.5 to −2.1 |
| SCC | 17,113 (86.0) | 85.5–86.4 | 15,504 (75.8) | 75.2–76.4 | −3.0 | −3.2 to −2.1 |
| ACA | 2,797 (14.0) | 13.6–14.5 | 4,952 (24.2) | 23.6–24.8 | 0.6 | 0.2–1.0 |

N number of cases, CI confidence interval, SCC squamous cell carcinoma, ACA adenocarcinoma, EAPC estimated annual percent change

Likewise an increased incidence of cervical adenocarcinoma has been noted in Europe [4, 10]. The rise in incidence of cervical adenocarcinoma including adenosquamous carcinoma has been particularly noted in younger women in countries with well-established screening programs [4, 5, 8, 11]. Interestingly, the most recent data suggest that levels are universally plateauing or even declining in the later years of data, suggesting improved detection (or possibly changes in epidemiologic drivers such as hormone use) may be having an effect on disease prevalence [12].

Racial and ethnic differences in the incidence of cervical adenocarcinoma have been identified. Analysis of SEER data from 1976 to 2000 showed that the incidence of cervical adenocarcinoma rose linearly with age in African-American women while the incidence plateaued in white women [8]. Recent analysis of SEER data (1998–2002) has demonstrated higher rates of adenocarcinoma in white women than in African-American women and in Hispanic women as compared to non-Hispanic women [13].

The rate of precursor squamous lesions far outweighs that of glandular lesions of the cervix in most series [14–17]. The SEER registry kept track of in situ carcinomas separately from invasive carcinomas from 1976 to 1995; thereafter, in situ and invasive carcinomas were grouped as one category. During that time period, of the 149,178 women with cervical carcinoma, 96 % were squamous lesions and 4 %

were glandular lesions; of the total, 121,793 (82 %) were in situ lesions. Of the in situ lesions, 99 % were squamous cell carcinoma in situ and only 1 % were AIS [18]. The data also showed that AIS increased at a steady rate in both white and African-American women during this period with the pace being greatest for white women [8]. Unlike squamous cell carcinoma, the incidence of invasive adenocarcinoma is greater than that of AIS [18]. Studies have suggested that screening is less effective in detection of endocervical adeno-carcinoma [19, 20]. Wang et al., in an analysis of SEER data from 1976 to 1995, noted in white women that the in situ-to-invasive ratio for squamous cell carcinoma rose from 2.25 to 6.69 (threefold) while that for adenocarcinoma rose from 0.2 to 0.8 (fourfold) [8]. In both tumor types, the reason for these increases of in situ versus invasive tumors is almost certainly better detection as well as potentially an increased preva-lence. In a retrospective study of cases from large Australian cytology laboratories, the sensitivity for detection of AIS in cytology samples was found to be up to 54.3 % [21].

# Etiology of Endocervical Adenocarcinoma and AIS

Almost all cervical squamous cell carcinomas are associated with high risk human papillomavirus (hrHPV) [22–24]. Endocervical adenocarcinoma is also associated with hrHPV but the prevalence is somewhat lower, approximately 90 % [25–28]. Endocervical adenocarcinomas positive for hrHPV are predominantly of the usual type which make up about 80 % of all endocervical adenocarcinomas [29]. The presumed precursor lesion of the usual type, AIS is positive for hrHPV in nearly 100 % of cases [28]. Although less commonly found in squamous lesions of the cervix, HPV18 and its associated type 45 are identified in a substantial number of in situ and invasive adenocarcinomas. HPV16 is also very commonly identified, but is not in the majority as is noted in squamous lesions [17, 25, 28, 30, 31]. Recently the Asian American variant of HPV16 has been preferentially associated with glandular neoplasia. It has been suggested that this variant is more prone to cause effects in the estrogen-associated areas of the host genome in line with the data that shows that hormone use may be more commonly associated with glandular carcinogenesis [28, 30–35]. The type of HPV present has not been found to impact survival in women with endocervical adenocarcinoma [31].

The epidemiologic risk factors for the development of the most common forms of endocervical adenocarcinoma are similar to squamous cell carcinoma and are those associated with sexually transmitted disease: use of oral contraceptives, multiple sexual partners, and young age at first intercourse [23]. Unlike squamous cell carcinoma, cigarette smoking is not associated with increased risk of endocervical adenocarcinoma. Unlike squamous cell carcinoma, endocervical adenocarcinoma appears to be less commonly associated with high parity but has a greater association with obesity (which is a known cause of increased endogenous estrogen production) [32]. Exogenous hormone use also has been shown to be a factor in the development of glandular cancers [11, 20, 36].

## Clinical Features of Endocervical Adenocarcinoma and AIS

In women with early stage tumors, endocervical adenocarcinoma may be asymptomatic or may present with abnormal vaginal bleeding (irregular, heavy, or postcoital) [33, 37, 38]. More advanced tumors may present with pelvic or low back pain. Depending on the type of adenocarcinoma present, up to 50 % of patients will have a visible tumor mass on physical exam [33]. Deeply infiltrative tumors can cause a diffusely enlarged, barrel-shaped cervix. The absence of a grossly identifiable tumor may correspond to an early stage tumor or if higher stage, to a deeply invasive tumor high in the endocervical canal [38].

AIS of the cervix is almost always asymptomatic with no lesion detectable on physical examination. AIS most commonly arises at the transformation zone and therefore colposcopic abnormalities may be visible. It is generally unifocal, but in some cases it can be discontinuous with additional foci present elsewhere in the endocervical canal.

# Diagnosis of Endocervical Neoplasia

In patients who are symptomatic or who have a grossly visible mass, a biopsy is performed. The type of biopsy (cervical biopsy, endocervical curettage, or endometrial biopsy) depends on the clinical scenario.

In asymptomatic patients, cervical cancer screening by cytology plays a major role in diagnosis. The accuracy of screening for glandular neoplasia by cervical cytology will be discussed in Chap. 2; however, it can be stated that the majority of women with glandular neoplasia of the cervix will have abnormal cytology. Up to 88 % of women with endocervical adenocarcinoma and the majority of those with AIS will have an abnormal Pap test [38–41].

According to the American Society for Colposcopy and Cervical Pathology (ASCCP), 2012 guidelines for management of women with cytologic abnormalities and cervical cancer precursors, the work-up will differ depending on the type and degree of abnormal cytology interpretation [42]. The recommended management for women with a cytologic interpretation of atypical glandular cells, AIS, and adenocarcinoma is colposcopy with endocervical curettage (ECC). Triage by reflex hrHPV testing is not recommended because the test does not identify women who need less aggressive work-up [42]. Endometrial sampling is added if the patient is older than 35 years. If atypical endometrial cells are identified, the work-up begins with endometrial and endocervical sampling and will proceed to colposcopy only if no endometrial pathology is found. If the atypical glandular cells are favored to be neoplastic or a firm cytologic diagnosis of AIS or adenocarcinoma has been made but the initial biopsies are negative for invasive disease, an excisional biopsy (loop electrosurgical excision procedure or cold knife cone) followed by ECC is recommended [42]. Review and confirmation of the original cytologic interpretation is recommended if an excisional procedure is being contemplated.

# References

1. Kurman RJ, Solomon D. The Bethesda system for reporting cervical/vaginal cytologic diagnoses. New York: Springer; 1994.
2. Solomon D, Nayar R. The Bethesda System for reporting cervical cytology. New York: Springer; 2004.
3. Mikuta JJ, Celebre JA. Adenocarcinoma of the cervix. Obstet Gynecol. 1969;33(6):753–6.
4. Vizcaino AP, Moreno V, Bosch FX, Munoz N, Barros-Dios XM, Parkin DM. International trends in the incidence of cervical cancer: I. Adenocarcinoma and adenosquamous cell carcinomas. Int J Cancer. 1998;75(4):536–45.
5. Bulk S, Visser O, Rozendaal L, Verheijen RH, Meijer CJ. Cervical cancer in the Netherlands 1989-1998: decrease of squamous cell carcinoma in older women, increase of adenocarcinoma in younger women. Int J Cancer. 2005;113(6):1005–9.
6. Smith HO, Tiffany MF, Qualls CR, Key CR. The rising incidence of adenocarcinoma relative to squamous cell carcinoma of the uterine cervix in the United States—a 24-year population-based study. Gynecol Oncol. 2000;78(2):97–105.
7. Ward KK, Shah NR, Saenz CC, McHale MT, Alvarez EA, Plaxe SC. Changing demographics of cervical cancer in the United States (1973-2008). Gynecol Oncol. 2012;126(3):330–3.
8. Wang SS, Sherman ME, Hildesheim A, Lacey Jr JV, Devesa S. Cervical adenocarcinoma and squamous cell carcinoma incidence trends among white women and black women in the United States for 1976-2000. Cancer. 2004;100(5):1035–44.
9. Sherman ME, Wang SS, Carreon J, Devesa SS. Mortality trends for cervical squamous and adenocarcinoma in the United States. Relation to incidence and survival. Cancer. 2005;103(6): 1258–64.
10. Bray F, Carstensen B, Moller H, Zappa M, Zakelj MP, Lawrence G, et al. Incidence trends of adenocarcinoma of the cervix in 13 European countries. Cancer Epidemiol Biomarkers Prev. 2005;14(9):2191–9.

11. Zaino RJ. Symposium part I: adenocarcinoma in situ, glandular dysplasia, and early invasive adenocarcinoma of the uterine cervix. Int J Gynecol Pathol. 2002;21(4):314–26.

12. Mathew A, George PS. Trends in incidence and mortality rates of squamous cell carcinoma and adenocarcinoma of cervix—worldwide. Asian Pac J Cancer Prev. 2009;10(4):645–50.

13. Saraiya M, Ahmed F, Krishnan S, Richards TB, Unger ER, Lawson HW. Cervical cancer incidence in a prevaccine era in the United States, 1998-2002. Obstet Gynecol. 2007;109(2 Pt 1): 360–70.

14. Mount SL, Papillo JL. A study of 10,296 pediatric and adolescent Papanicolaou smear diagnoses in northern New England. Pediatrics. 1999;103(3):539–45.

15. Insinga RP, Glass AG, Rush BB. Diagnoses and outcomes in cervical cancer screening: a population-based study. Am J Obstet Gynecol. 2004;191(1):105–13.

16. Benard VB, Eheman CR, Lawson HW, Blackman DK, Anderson C, Helsel W, et al. Cervical screening in the National Breast and Cervical Cancer Early Detection Program, 1995-2001. Obstet Gynecol. 2004;103(3):564–71.

17. Wright Jr TC, Stoler MH, Behrens CM, Apple R, Derion T, Wright TL. The ATHENA human papillomavirus study: design, methods, and baseline results. Am J Obstet Gynecol. 2012; 206(1):46.e1–11.

18. Plaxe SC, Saltzstein SL. Estimation of the duration of the preclinical phase of cervical adenocarcinoma suggests that there is ample opportunity for screening. Gynecol Oncol. 1999;75(1):55–61.

19. Mitchell H, Medley G, Gordon I, Giles G. Cervical cytology reported as negative and risk of adenocarcinoma of the cervix: no strong evidence of benefit. Br J Cancer. 1995;71(4):894–7.

20. Nieminen P, Kallio M, Hakama M. The effect of mass screening on incidence and mortality of squamous and adenocarcinoma of cervix uteri. Obstet Gynecol. 1995;85(6):1017–21.

21. Schoolland M, Segal A, Allpress S, Miranda A, Frost FA, Sterrett GF. Adenocarcinoma in situ of the cervix. Cancer. 2002; 96(6):330–7.

22. Walboomers JM, Jacobs MV, Manos MM, Bosch FX, Kummer JA, Shah KV, et al. Human papillomavirus is a necessary cause of invasive cervical cancer worldwide. J Pathol. 1999; 189(1):12–9.

23. Castellsague X, Diaz M, de Sanjose S, Munoz N, Herrero R, Franceschi S, et al. Worldwide human papillomavirus etiology of

cervical adenocarcinoma and its cofactors: implications for screening and prevention. J Natl Cancer Inst. 2006;98(5): 303–15.

24. Li N, Franceschi S, Howell-Jones R, Snijders PJ, Clifford GM. Human papillomavirus type distribution in 30,848 invasive cervical cancers worldwide: variation by geographical region, histological type and year of publication. Int J Cancer. 2011; 128(4):927–35.

25. Pirog EC, Kleter B, Olgac S, Bobkiewicz P, Lindeman J, Quint WG, et al. Prevalence of human papillomavirus DNA in different histological subtypes of cervical adenocarcinoma. Am J Pathol. 2000;157(4):1055–62.

26. Andersson S, Rylander E, Larsson B, Strand A, Silfversvard C, Wilander E. The role of human papillomavirus in cervical adeno-carcinoma carcinogenesis. Eur J Cancer. 2001;37(2):246–50.

27. Clifford G, Franceschi S. Members of the human papillomavirus type 18 family (alpha-7 species) share a common association with adenocarcinoma of the cervix. Int J Cancer. 2008;122(7):1684–5.

28. Quint KD, de Koning MN, Geraets DT, Quint WG, Pirog EC. Comprehensive analysis of human papillomavirus and Chlamydia trachomatis in in-situ and invasive cervical adenocar-cinoma. Gynecol Oncol. 2009;114(3):390–4.

29. Young RH, Clement PB. Endocervical adenocarcinoma and its variants: their morphology and differential diagnosis. Histopathology. 2002;41(3):185–207.

30. An HJ, Kim KR, Kim IS, Kim DW, Park MH, Park IA, et al. Prevalence of human papillomavirus DNA in various histologi-cal subtypes of cervical adenocarcinoma: a population-based study. Mod Pathol. 2005;18(4):528–34.

31. Baalbergen A, Smedts F, Ewing P, Snijders PJ, Meijer CJ, Helmerhorst TJ. HPV-type has no impact on survival of patients with adenocarcinoma of the uterine cervix. Gynecol Oncol. 2013; 128:530–4.

32. Appleby P, Beral V, Berrington de Gonzalez A, Colin D, Franceschi S, Goodill A, et al. Carcinoma of the cervix and tobacco smoking: collaborative reanalysis of individual data on 13,541 women with carcinoma of the cervix and 23,017 women without carcinoma of the cervix from 23 epidemiological studies. Int J Cancer. 2006;118(6):1481–95.

33. Hurt WG, Silverberg SG, Frable WJ, Belgrad R, Crooks LD. Adenocarcinoma of the cervix: histopathologic and clinical features. Am J Obstet Gynecol. 1977;129(3):304–15.

34. Ostor AG, Duncan A, Quinn M, Rome R. Adenocarcinoma in situ of the uterine cervix: an experience with 100 cases. Gynecol Oncol. 2000;79(2):207–10.

35. Wright Jr TC, Massad LS, Dunton CJ, Spitzer M, Wilkinson EJ, Solomon D. 2006 consensus guidelines for the management of women with cervical intraepithelial neoplasia or adenocarcinoma in situ. Am J Obstet Gynecol. 2007;197(4):340–5.

36. Schoolland M, Allpress S, Sterrett GF. Adenocarcinoma of the cervix. Cancer. 2002;96(1):5–13.

37. Shingleton HM, Gore H, Bradley DH, Soong SJ. Adenocarcinoma of the cervix. I. Clinical evaluation and pathologic features. Am J Obstet Gynecol. 1981;139(7):799–814.

38. Saigo PE, Cain JM, Kim WS, Gaynor JJ, Johnson K, Lewis Jr JL. Prognostic factors in adenocarcinoma of the uterine cervix. Cancer. 1986;57(8):1584–93.

39. Mulvany N, Ostor A. Microinvasive adenocarcinoma of the cervix: a cytohistopathologic study of 40 cases. Diagn Cytopathol. 1997;16(5):430–6.

40. Ostor AG. Early invasive adenocarcinoma of the uterine cervix. Int J Gynecol Pathol. 2000;19(1):29–38.

41. Tobon H, Dave H. Adenocarcinoma in situ of the cervix. Clinicopathologic observations of 11 cases. Int J Gynecol Pathol. 1988;7(2):139–51.

42. Massad LS, Einstein MH, Huh WK, Katki HA, Kinney WK, Schiffman M, et al. 2012 updated consensus guidelines for the management of abnormal cervical cancer screening tests and cancer precursors. J Low Genit Tract Dis. 2013;17(5 Suppl 1):S1–27.

# Chapter 2
# Processing, Reporting, and Sensitivity of Cervical Cytology with an Emphasis on Glandular Lesions

## Obtaining the Cervical Cytology Sample

Identification of glandular lesions in cervical cytology begins with an adequate sampling of the cervical transformation zone and endocervical canal. This is achieved by performance of a speculum examination of the cervix which entails opening of the vaginal canal with a speculum in order to visualize the ectocervix and cervical os. Cells are obtained from the exposed external cervix, the ectocervix, and from the endocervical canal, in order to assure evaluation of the transformation zone, the area of highest risk for preneoplastic and neoplastic squamous and glandular lesions. Several devices are available for cytology sampling. Cotton/dacron swabs had been widely used in the past but have been found to fail to release abnormal cells for examination so their use is no longer recommended [1]. Wooden spatulas should not be used with liquid-based fixatives, but may be used to make direct smears. Currently the most commonly used devices are the plastic spatula, the endocervical brush, and the cervical broom (Fig. 2.1). All devices are intended to circumferentially scrape the cervix. When using the endocervical brush, the bristles nearest the operator should be at the level of the external os of the cervix in order to obtain the best sample; the brush should be rotated 90–180° in one direction being

R.H. Tambouret and D.C. Wilbur, *Glandular Lesions of the Uterine Cervix*, Essentials in Cytopathology 19, DOI 10.1007/978-1-4939-1989-5_2, © Springer Science+Business Media New York 2015

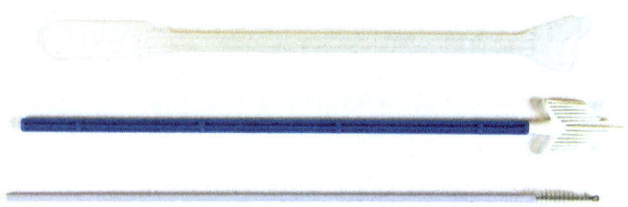

FIG. 2.1 Devices used to obtain a cervical cytology sample: Plastic spatula (*top*), Cervical broom (*center*) and Endocervical brush (*bottom*)

careful not to over-rotate. The use of both the plastic spatula for the ectocervix and the endocervical brush for the endocervix has been shown to provide more endocervical cells than the spatula alone [2]. The cervix broom is a device designed to sample both the ecto- and endocervix simultaneously. The central longer bristles are inserted into the endocervical canal while the shorter, more peripheral bristles are splayed over the ectocervix. The bristles of the broom are angled in such a way that an adequate sample can only be obtained if the broom is turned *clockwise* for 360° five times.

For conventional smears (CS), the cell samples are smeared from the spatula (either wooden or plastic) and rolled from the brush onto a glass slide and immediately fixed in alcohol, either by direct immersion into a solution of ethanol or by the use of aerosol spray fixation (Fig. 2.2). The CS is now ready for staining with the Papanicolaou (Pap) stain, the stain mandated by the Clinical Laboratory Improvement Amendment of 1988. The Pap stain uses hematoxylin to color the nucleus and several other colors to stain the cytoplasm. The stain was originally developed to analyze the degree of keratinization of the squamous cell cytoplasm but also adequately stains endocervical cells.

Alternatively, the sampling device (only plastic) can be directly immersed into a proprietary vial of alcohol-based fixative in order to capture and release the cells; this method constitutes "liquid-based cytology" (LBC). In North America,

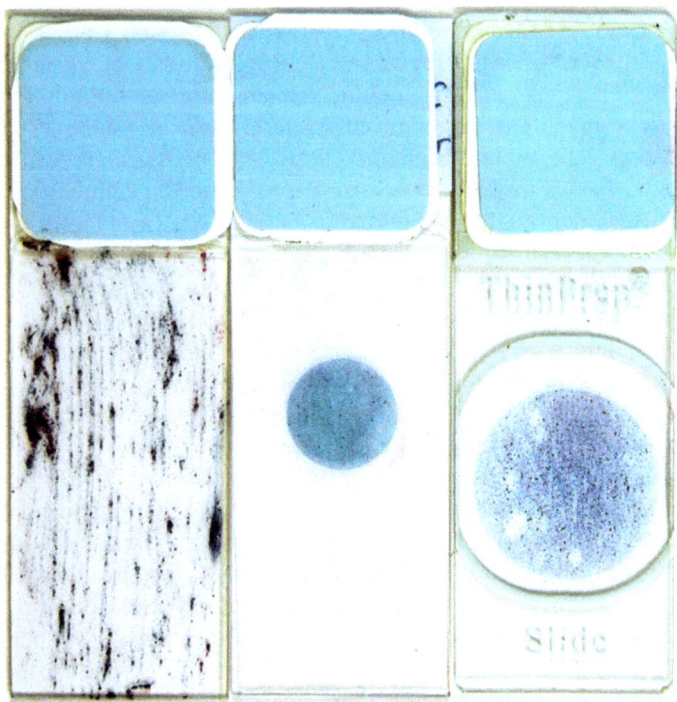

Fig. 2.2  Slide preparations used for cervical cytology: Conventional smear (*left*), SurePath™ (*center*) and ThinPrep® (*right*)

two types of LBC are commercially available: ThinPrep® Pap Test (Hologic, Inc., Marlborough, MA) and BD SurePath™ Pap Test (Becton-Dickinson) (Fig. 2.2). The tests have features that produce subtle but important differences in cervical cytology, especially relative to glandular epithelium.

ThinPrep (TP) employs a methanol-based fixative. The clinician must vigorously agitate the sampling device to extract the maximum amount of cells prior to removing and discarding the device. SurePath (SP) uses an ethanol-based fixative of relatively low concentration. The sampling devices used with SP have detachable heads which are simply dropped into the fixative.

Sample processing differs for the two products leading to a different presentation of the sample on the cytology slide. The TP sample is drawn up through a membrane without any preliminary extraction of unwanted material (mucus, red blood cells, or leukocytes) to which the cells adhere while fluid passes through to be discarded. When the cellularity is sufficient, the cells are pressed to a glass slide. The TP process gives the cell sample a relatively flattened presentation on the slide. SP processing begins with centrifugation with density gradient material to remove excess blood and leukocytes. An aliquot of sample is then allowed to settle by force of gravity onto the slide producing a more three-dimensional quality to the presentation especially prominent in tightly cohesive groups of glandular cells.

The decision to use CS vs. LBC depends on several factors including the rate of fully adequate samples, the reliability of the screening process, the ability to perform additional concurrent tests, and the cost. The cost of LBC is more than CS due to the need for disposables and additional laboratory equipment which is mitigated when additional tests are performed as a second separate sample is unnecessary for the other tests. Despite these differences between CS and LBC, the American College of Obstetricians and Gynecologists does not advocate for one method over the other citing a meta-analysis report of eight studies and a randomized trial that failed to show a significant difference [3–5]. Regarding the unsatisfactory rates between TP and SP, a recent systematic review and meta-analysis of 14 SP studies and 28 TP studies found significantly fewer unsatisfactory SP samples as compared to TP [6].

Performance of CS as compared to LBC has not found significant differences in the rate of detection of high grade squamous intraepithelial lesions [5, 7–9]. On the other hand, observational studies suggest that CS does not perform as well as LBC in the detection of glandular abnormalities [7, 10–14].

Obscuring blood may result in an unsatisfactory CS sample so the first few days of the menstrual cycle should be avoided [15]. Appropriately processed LBC and HPV testing results do not appear to be affected by the timing of the menstrual cycle [16]. Likewise gel lubricant on the speculum does not appear to interfere with the cytology [17, 18].

## The Requisition

The cervical cytology sample must be accompanied by a requisition form which should be completed by the clinician in order to provide the basic patient information needed to interpret the sample. Required elements by US Federal Regulations include patient name, age, date of birth, ordering clinician, and whether the patient is undergoing routine screening or is at high risk for cervical disease. The most important elements for the specific cytologic evaluation of glandular cells are the patient's age, the last menstrual period, gestational history, use of an intrauterine device (IUD) as a method of contraception, history of diethylstilbestrol exposure in utero, and any history of prior abnormal cytology samples or gynecologic pathology (Table 2.1). During the analysis of the slide, the cytologist should correlate the cytologic findings with the clinical information provided. If a discrepancy is identified between the information provided and the cytologic findings, the cytologist must make an attempt to explain the differences. If the electronic medical record and laboratory information system are available, the records can be searched for clarification. As an example, changes in glandular cells suggestive of the presence of an IUD may be

TABLE 2.1 The cytology requisition form

| |
| --- |
| Patient demographics: Name; Age; Date of Birth; Medical record number |
| Date of procedure |
| Ordering Clinician |
| Sample obtained for : routine screening; follow-up of high risk |
| Patient history: gestational history; last menstrual period; contraception; other history |

identified, but the clinician has not indicated the placement of an IUD. Not infrequently in searching the medical record the history of IUD placement will be found.

# Image Analysis-Assisted Screening

Screening of cervical cytology slides is often assisted by image analysis (also known as automated review) prior to the review by the cytotechnologist. Two systems are FDA approved and available for image analysis: the ThinPrep Imager (TPI) and the SurePath FocalPoint family (Slide Profiler, Guided System [GS] and Location Guided Screening (LGS)) of which the GS is nearly exclusively used in North America. Both systems (TPI and FP GS) evaluate LBC slides and select fields of view (FOV) most likely to harbor abnormal cells for presentation to the cytotechnologist for initial review. The FOV make up approximately one third of the total slide area for both devices. If cytologic abnormalities are not identified by the cytotechnologist on initial review, the case is signed out as negative. If a potential abnormality is identified, the full slide is manually screened by the cytotechnologist. Both systems rely on robotic instrumentation that incorporates automated microscopy with high-speed image analysis. Both systems use complex computer algorithms to analyze morphologic findings. At the heart of the ThinPrep system is the use of a modified "Feulgen-like" hematoxylin stain which enables the image analysis software to calculate the relative stoichiometric DNA content of the epithelial cells. FOVs are presented in a geographic fashion for each slide. The FocalPoint family uses traditional Papanicolaou-stained slides and hierarchically "scores" each slide and the FOVs on each slide, presenting the FOVs to the reviewer in order of probability of abnormality (highest probability FOVs first). In addition, the slides within a given run are ranked according to their potential to harbor abnormal cells.

Both the TPI system and FP GS system have been found to accurately triage slides with glandular cells abnormalities to full manual review [19, 20]. However, as compared to the ranking of slides containing high grade squamous lesions (HSILs are routinely ranked at the highest scores), the FP GS system may not always assign a slide containing a glandular lesion to the highest scoring ranks (slides with glandular lesions can occur at any score level) and hence all slides need to be carefully reviewed for their presence [21].

# Specimen Reporting Format and Terminology for Reporting Glandular Lesions Identified on Cervical Cytology

In 1988 a new nomenclature, the Bethesda System (TBS), for reporting cervical cytology results was devised in order to standardize terminology, to produce clinically useful reports improving communication with clinicians and other cytologists, and to improve the reproducibility of diagnostic criteria for each entity. The Bethesda terminology has undergone one revision which took place at a second consensus conference in 2001. In the newest edition of the terminology, recommended components of the report include specimen type (conventional smear vs. LBC), adequacy (satisfactory or unsatisfactory), interpretation (negative for intraepithelial lesion or malignancy (NILM), other (endometrial cells in a woman over 40 years of age) or epithelial cell abnormalities (squamous or glandular) or other malignant neoplasms), ancillary testing, and automated review. An optional quality indicator component allows the report to signal features such as the absence of an endocervical/transformation zone component in an otherwise satisfactory sample, which may have clinical utility in selected circumstances. Under the interpretative category of NILM are included reactive changes; for example, reactive endocervical cells resulting from the presence of an intrauterine contraceptive device. Epithelial cell abnormalities: glandular are subcategorized according to cell-type (endocervical, endometrial, or extrauterine) and as to severity (atypical not otherwise specified, atypical favor neoplastic, adenocarcinoma in situ (AIS), and adenocarcinoma (ACA))

TABLE 2.2 Recommended Bethesda System cytology report format

SPECIMEN TYPE: CS vs. LBC
SPECIMEN ADEQUACY: Satisfactory vs. Unsatisfactory (Reason)
GENERAL CATEGORIZATION:
  Negative for intraepithelial lesion or malignancy (NILM)
  Other: See interpretation/result (e.g., endometrial cells in woman >40 years
  of age)
  Epithelial cell abnormality: Squamous vs. glandular
INTERPRETATION/RESULT:
  NILM: NOS or REACTIVE or ATROPHY or ORGANISMS
  SQUAMOUS CELL ABNORMALITIES
  GLANDULAR CELL ABNORMALITIES
    Atypical endocervical cell—NOS vs. favor neoplastic
    Atypical endometrial cells—NOS vs. favor neoplastic
    Atypical glandular cells—NOS vs. favor neoplastic
    Endocervical adenocarcinoma in situ
    Adenocarcinoma—endocervical vs. endometrial vs. extrauterine vs. NOS
  OTHER MALIGNANT NEOPLASMS
QUALITY INDICATORS: e.g., obscuring blood, no endocervical cells
ANCILLARY TESTING: HPV test method and result
AUTOMATED REVIEW: device and result

*CS* conventional smear, *LBC* liquid based cytology, *NOS* not otherwise
specified

(Table 2.2). The first edition of TBS used the umbrella term, atypical glandular cells (AGC) of undetermined significance (AGUS) and required qualification as to cell of origin (endocervical or endometrial). In the second edition, AGUS was abandoned for at the interpretive designation AGC.

Prior to the revised 2001 TBS, the presence of cytologically benign exfoliated endometrial cells out of phase (present in the second half of the menstrual cycle) were reported for women of all ages. However, because studies showed that in women less than 40 years of age, this finding was not found to harbor significant endometrial pathology when further investigated, the terminology was modified. Women aged 40 years or more are occasionally found to have endometrial neoplasia, and as such, reporting of benign-appearing endometrial cells is now restricted to women aged 40 years or older, and in practice is often further restricted to only postmenopausal or premenopausal women over 40 only if the endometrial cells are present in the second half of the menstrual cycle.

# Sensitivity of Cervical Cytology for the Presence of Glandular Abnormalities

Fewer studies concerning the sensitivity of cervical cytology for glandular abnormalities have been published than have been for the far more common squamous lesions. The problem of sensitivity has been approached in two ways, either as a retrospective review of patients with histologically diagnosed AIS/ACA or as a follow-up study of glandular lesions identified on cervical cytology.

Through follow-up studies the frequency of the cytologic diagnosis of AGUS or AGC has been found to vary from 0.11 to 0.46 % [12, 22–28]. Follow-up studies also permit determination of the rate of subsequent histologic abnormalities overall and by subcategorization of AGUS or AGC or by associated cytology findings.

The incidence of significant pathology following the AGUS or AGC interpretation varied widely, from as low as 9 % to as high as 58.6 % [29, 30] but almost all studies show a rate of over 20 % [23, 28, 31]. This level of variation may be due in part to uneven application of diagnostic criteria to the cytology sample. Subclassification of AGC as favor neoplasia results in a higher incidence of significant abnormalities on follow-up histology [28]. Association of AGC interpretation with a squamous lesion (ASCUS, ASC-H, LSIL, or HSIL) will more often be associated with a significant squamous lesion than a glandular lesion [25]. Interpretation of AGC in younger (<40 years) or premenopausal women is more likely to be associated with HSIL [25, 31].

Retrospective reviews of prior cytology following the diagnosis of adenocarcinoma in situ (AIS) or endocervical adenocarcinoma (ECA) on histology have provided insights into the sensitivity of cervical cytology for glandular lesions. By analyzing data from a cervical cytology registry in Australia, a retrospective review of ECA and AIS revealed several findings. The sensitivity of cervical cytology preceding the diagnosis of AIS was found to be about 50 % [32]. Examination of cytology samples preceding cases of ECA and AIS revealed a significant rate of sampling errors (22.2 % and 35 %, respectively) [33, 34]. Screening/interpretive errors accounted for 19.4 % of errors in cases of ECA and 10.4 % of AIS cases.

Another retrospective review of ECA found the sensitivity of a single cervical cytology between 45 and 76 % after review of the available smears [35]. The authors attributed a significant number of the false negatives to misinterpretation of preneoplastic/neoplastic glandular epithelium as normal lower uterine segment, tubal metaplasia or reactive endocervical cells. Other studies have noted a lower sensitivity for AIS or ECA when HSIL is also present [36]. The location of glandular neoplasia higher in the endocervical canal rather than at the transformation zone has been associated with a greater false negative rate for AIS [37].

The use of LBC rather than conventional smears has been associated with improved sensitivity for glandular lesions of the cervix [12, 23].

Certainly the move to new sampling devices that obtain more endocervical epithelium from higher in the canal has been found to be more sensitive in the detection of glandular lesions; however, increased recognition of the cytologic features of these processes undoubtedly also plays a role in sensitivity improvements that have been noted over time.

# References

1. Rubio CA. The false negative smear. II. The trapping effect of collecting instruments. Obstet Gynecol. 1977;49(5):576–80.
2. Marchand L, Mundt M, Klein G, Agarwal SC. Optimal collection technique and devices for a quality pap smear. WMJ. 2005; 104(6):51–5.
3. Practice Bulletin Number 131 A. Screening for cervical cancer. Obstet Gynecol. 2012;120:122–38.
4. Siebers AG, Klinkhamer PJ, Arbyn M, Raifu AO, Massuger LF, Bulten J. Cytologic detection of cervical abnormalities using liquid-based compared with conventional cytology: a randomized controlled trial. Obstet Gynecol. 2008;112(6):1327–34.
5. Arbyn M, Bergeron C, Klinkhamer P, Martin-Hirsch P, Siebers AG, Bulten J. Liquid compared with conventional cervical cytology:

a systematic review and meta-analysis. Obstet Gynecol. 2008;111(1):167–77.

6. Fontaine D, Narine N, Naugler C. Unsatisfactory rates vary between cervical cytology samples prepared using ThinPrep and SurePath platforms: a review and meta-analysis. BMJ Open. 2012;2(2):e000847.

7. Ronco G, Cuzick J, Pierotti P, Cariaggi MP, Dalla Palma P, Naldoni C, et al. Accuracy of liquid based versus conventional cytology: overall results of new technologies for cervical cancer screening: randomised controlled trial. BMJ. 2007;335(7609):28.

8. Davey E, Barratt A, Irwig L, Chan SF, Macaskill P, Mannes P, et al. Effect of study design and quality on unsatisfactory rates, cytology classifications, and accuracy in liquid-based versus conventional cervical cytology: a systematic review [see comment]. Lancet. 2006;367(9505):122–32.

9. Whitlock EP, Vesco KK, Eder M, Lin JS, Senger CA, Burda BU. Liquid-based cytology and human papillomavirus testing to screen for cervical cancer: a systematic review for the U.S. Preventive Services Task Force. Ann Intern Med. 2011;155(10):687–97; W214–5.

10. Lee KR, Darragh TM, Joste NE, Krane JF, Sherman ME, Hurley LB, et al. Atypical glandular cells of undetermined significance (AGUS): interobserver reproducibility in cervical smears and corresponding thin-layer preparations. Am J Clin Pathol. 2002;117(1):96–102.

11. Wang N, Emancipator SN, Rose P, Rodriguez M, Abdul-Karim FW. Histologic follow-up of atypical endocervical cells. Liquid-based, thin-layer preparation vs. conventional Pap smear. Acta Cytol. 2002;46(3):453–7.

12. Bai H, Sung CJ, Steinhoff MM. ThinPrep Pap Test promotes detection of glandular lesions of the endocervix. Diagn Cytopathol. 2000;23(1):19–22.

13. Hecht JL, Sheets EE, Lee KR. Atypical glandular cells of undetermined significance in conventional cervical/vaginal smears and thin-layer preparations. Cancer. 2002;96(1):1–4.

14. Burnley C, Dudding N, Parker M, Parsons P, Whitaker CJ, Young W. Glandular neoplasia and borderline endocervical reporting rates before and after conversion to the SurePath(TM) liquid-based cytology (LBC) system. Diagn Cytopathol. 2011;39(12): 869–74.

15. Vooijs GP, van der Graaf Y, Elias AG. Cellular composition of cervical smears in relation to the day of the menstrual cycle and the method of contraception. Acta Cytol. 1987;31(4):417–26.

16. Sherman ME, Carreon JD, Schiffman M. Performance of cytology and human papillomavirus testing in relation to the menstrual cycle. Br J Cancer. 2006;94(11):1690–6.

17. Amies AM, Miller L, Lee SK, Koutsky L. The effect of vaginal speculum lubrication on the rate of unsatisfactory cervical cytology diagnosis. Obstet Gynecol. 2002;100(5 Pt 1):889–92.

18. Griffith WF, Stuart GS, Gluck KL, Heartwell SF. Vaginal speculum lubrication and its effects on cervical cytology and microbiology. Contraception. 2005;72(1):60–4.

19. Bowditch RC, Clarke JM, Baird PJ, Greenberg ML. Results of an Australian trial using SurePath liquid-based cervical cytology with FocalPoint computer-assisted screening technology. Diagn Cytopathol. 2012;40(12):1093–9.

20. Friedlander MA, Rudomina D, Lin O. Effectiveness of the Thin Prep Imaging System in the detection of adenocarcinoma of the gynecologic system. Cancer. 2008;114(1):7–12.

21. Chute DJ, Lim H, Kong CS. BD focalpoint slide profiler performance with atypical glandular cells on SurePath Papanicolaou smears. Cancer Cytopathol. 2010;118(2):68–74.

22. Ashfaq R, Gibbons D, Vela C, Saboorian MH, Iliya F. ThinPrep Pap Test. Accuracy for glandular disease. Acta Cytol. 1999;43(1): 81–5.

23. Schorge JO, Hossein Saboorian M, Hynan L, Ashfaq R. ThinPrep detection of cervical and endometrial adenocarcinoma: a retrospective cohort study. Cancer. 2002;96(6):338–43.

24. Adhya AK, Mahesha V, Srinivasan R, Nijhawan R, Rajwanshi A, Suri V, et al. Atypical glandular cells in cervical smears: histological correlation and a suggested plan of management based on age of the patient in a low-resource setting. Cytopathology. 2009; 20(6):375–9.

25. Zhao C, Austin RM, Pan J, Barr N, Martin SE, Raza A, et al. Clinical significance of atypical glandular cells in conventional pap smears in a large, high-risk U.S. west coast minority population. Acta Cytol. 2009;53(2):153–9.

26. Goff BA, Atanasoff P, Brown E, Muntz HG, Bell DA, Rice LW. Endocervical glandular atypia in Papanicolaou smears. Obstet Gynecol. 1992;79(1):101–4.

27. Schnatz PF, Guile M, O'Sullivan DM, Sorosky JI. Clinical significance of atypical glandular cells on cervical cytology. Obstet Gynecol. 2006;107(3):701–8.

28. DeSimone CP, Day ME, Tovar MM, Dietrich 3rd CS, Eastham ML, Modesitt SC. Rate of pathology from atypical glandular cell

Pap tests classified by the Bethesda 2001 nomenclature. Obstet Gynecol. 2006;107(6):1285–91.

29. Sharpless KE, Schnatz PF, Mandavilli S, Greene JF, Sorosky JI. Dysplasia associated with atypical glandular cells on cervical cytology. Obstet Gynecol. 2005;105(3):494–500.

30. Valdini A, Vaccaro C, Pechinsky G, Abernathy V. Incidence and evaluation of an AGUS Papanicolaou smear in primary care. J Am Board Fam Pract. 2001;14(3):172–7.

31. Duska LR, Flynn CF, Chen A, Whall-Strojwas D, Goodman A. Clinical evaluation of atypical glandular cells of undetermined significance on cervical cytology. Obstet Gynecol. 1998;91(2): 278–82.

32. Schoolland M, Segal A, Allpress S, Miranda A, Frost FA, Sterrett GF. Adenocarcinoma in situ of the cervix. Cancer. 2002;96(6):330–7.

33. Schoolland M, Allpress S, Sterrett GF. Adenocarcinoma of the cervix. Cancer. 2002;96(1):5–13.

34. Ruba S, Schoolland M, Allpress S, Sterrett G. Adenocarcinoma in situ of the uterine cervix: screening and diagnostic errors in Papanicolaou smears. Cancer. 2004;102(5):280–7.

35. Krane JF, Granter SR, Trask CE, Hogan CL, Lee KR. Papanicolaou smear sensitivity for the detection of adenocarcinoma of the cervix: a study of 49 cases. Cancer. 2001;93(1): 8–15.

36. van Aspert-van Erp AJ, Smedts FM, Vooijs GP. Severe cervical glandular cell lesions with coexisting squamous cell lesions. Cancer. 2004;102(4):218–27.

37. Kalir T, Simsir A, Demopoulos HB, Demopoulos RI. Obstacles to the early detection of endocervical adenocarcinoma. Int J Gynecol Pathol. 2005;24(4):399–403.

# Chapter 3
# Normal Histology and Cytology of the Endocervix and Endometrium

An understanding of normal cervical and uterine glandular histology and cytology will aid in the recognition of glandular lesions in cervical cytology.

## Histology of the Normal Endocervix

The uterus, an inverted triangular shaped muscular organ with a central mucosal lined cavity, is divided into regions: the fundus, the corpus, the isthmus or lower uterine segment, and the endocervical canal and the exocervix (Fig. 3.1). The fallopian tubes enter the uterine cavity at the cornua of the uterus. Distally, the cervix merges with the vagina. The internal os marks the boundary between the corpus and the endocervix. In the nulliparous woman, the cervix usually measures 3–4 cm in diameter and is approximately the same length as the corpus, but following childbearing the ratio of cervical length to corpus is approximately 1–2. Deep clefts created by invaginations of the endocervical epithelium into the stroma create the rugae characteristic of the endocervical canal. The clefts appear as glands on histologic sections but are not true glands. The endocervical canal transforms to the exocervix at the external os.

R.H. Tambouret and D.C. Wilbur, *Glandular Lesions of the Uterine Cervix*, Essentials in Cytopathology 19, DOI 10.1007/978-1-4939-1989-5_3,
© Springer Science+Business Media New York 2015

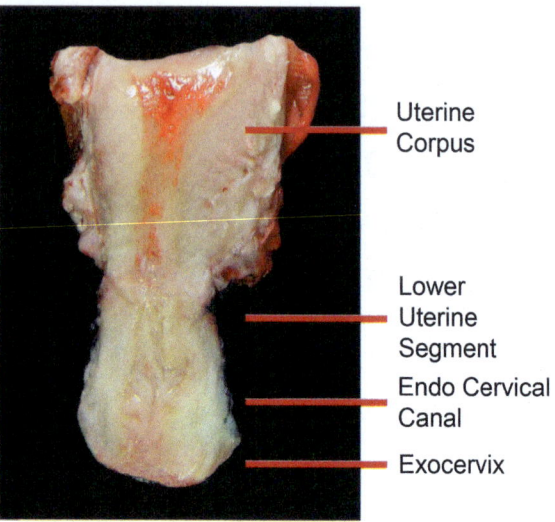

Uterine
Corpus

Lower
Uterine
Segment

Endo Cervical
Canal

Exocervix

FIG. 3.1  Uterus bivalved to reveal major landmarks: corpus, lower uterine segment, endocervical canal, and exocervix

The exocervix or ectocervix protrudes into the vagina and is known as the portio vaginalis. The exocervix is covered by non-cornified stratified squamous epithelium identical to the squamous epithelium covering the vagina (Fig. 3.2). A sharp demarcation between the squamous epithelium of the exocervix and the glandular epithelium of the endocervix is present either on the exocervix or in the endocervical canal depending on the reproductive age. Shortly after birth the squamo-columnar junction is found in the endocervical canal. At puberty, the squamo-columnar junction shifts to the exocervix where the exposed endocervical mucosa appears red and is known as ectropion. Gradually the exposed, more fragile glandular covering of the ectropion is replaced by more robust squamous epithelium through the process of squamous metaplasia, creating a new, functional squamo-columnar junction. The region between the original squamo-columnar junction and the functional squamo-columnar junction, where the surface endocervical epithelium has been replaced by

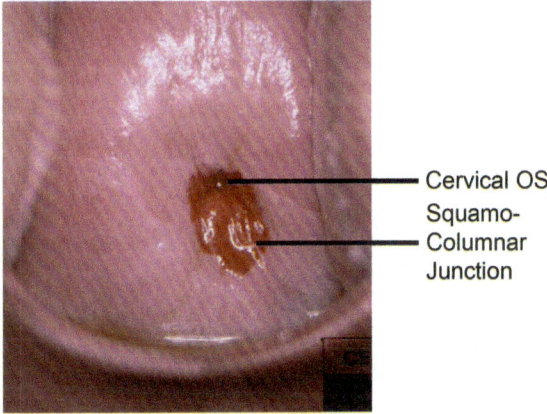

Cervical OS
Squamo-
Columnar
Junction

FIG. 3.2  Cervix as seen with the aid of a colposcope

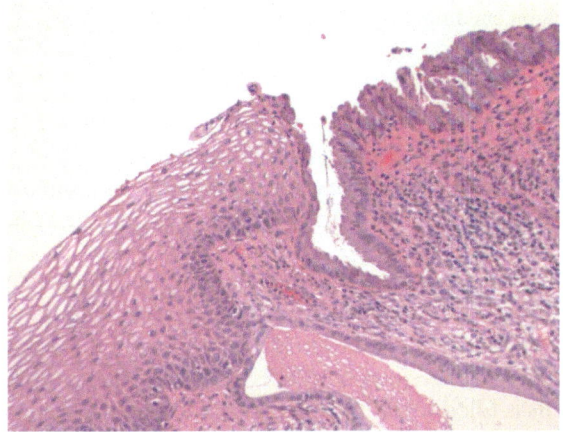

FIG. 3.3  Squamo-columnar junction of the transformation zone: junction of stratified squamous epithelium and endocervical epithelium; low magnification, hematoxylin and eosin stain

squamous epithelium, is known as the transformation zone and on histology can be recognized by the endocervical glands or clefts beneath the surface squamous epithelium (Fig. 3.3). The transformation zone is the region in which cervical squamous

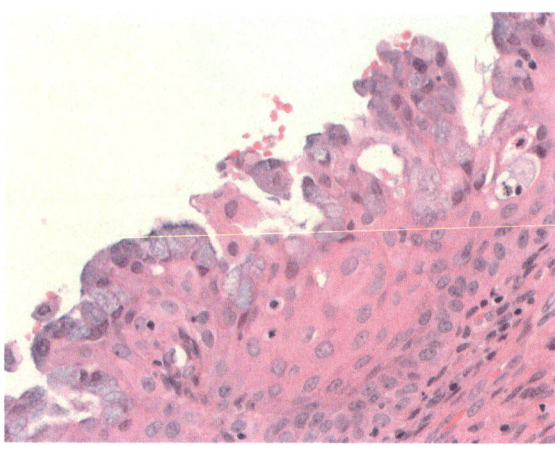

FIG. 3.4 Squamous metaplasia at the transformation zone: immature squamous metaplasia forms beneath the endocervical mucinous epithelium; medium magnification, hematoxylin and eosin stain

metaplasia arises from the reserve cells (Fig. 3.4). On histologic sections these immature metaplastic cells appear to undermine the residual endocervical epithelium. After menopause the functional transformation zone recedes into the endocervical canal.

The endocervical epithelium, comprises a single layer of predominantly mucin-secreting cells with small, usually basally placed nuclei, lines both the surface of the endocervical canal and the clefts or glands (Fig. 3.5). The cytoplasm of the cells is filled with fine mucin droplets and has a characteristic pale blue hue with the hematoxylin and eosin stain. Scattered nonsecretory ciliated cells are interspersed among the more numerous mucinous cells, presumably to propel the mucus expelled by the mucinous cells. The nuclei of the endocervical cells are round to slightly elongate with inapparent nucleoli when the cells are in the resting state. Injury or other stimuli will cause nucleoli to become prominent in enlarged nuclei. Mitotic figures are uncommon in nonneoplastic endocervical cells, but can be present in regenerative states.

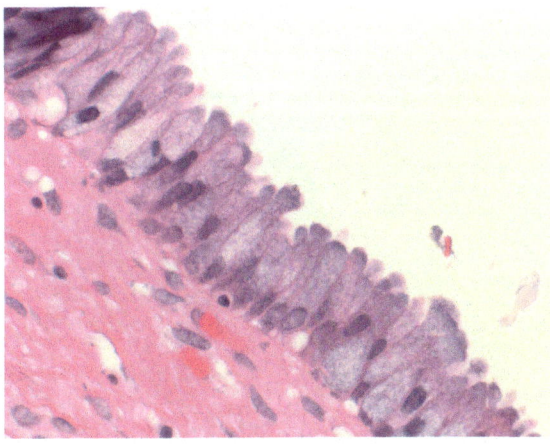

Fig. 3.5  Endocervical epithelium: a single layer of columnar cells with uniformly mucinous cytoplasm and small nuclei positioned near the cell attachment to the basement membrane; high magnification, hematoxylin and eosin stain

## Cytology of the Normal Endocervix

On cytology slides, normal endocervical glandular epithelium shows variable appearances depending on several factors: patient age and hormonal status, the level sampled within the endocervical canal, the sampling device, and the cytology preparation. Endocervical cells most commonly present as columnar cells, either singly or in variably sized groups, without attached stroma (Fig. 3.6). When displayed in profile, the single endocervical cell is recognized by the approximately twice longer than wide shape. The nucleus is round with a smooth or slightly irregular nuclear membrane contour and is located at the basal pole of the columnar cells. Small nucleoli may be identified within finely dispersed chromatin. The nuclear size can vary from slightly larger than a red blood cell to greater than the size of a polymorphonuclear leukocyte. Multinucleated endocervical cells are commonly encountered. Small dark knuckles protruding from the nuclear membrane into the cytoplasm have been described in association

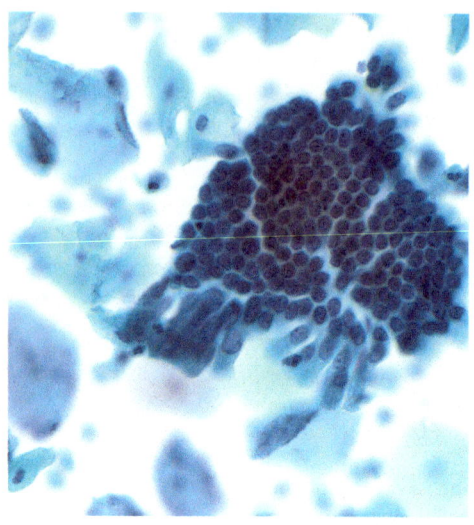

FIG. 3.6 Endocervical cells arranged mainly in honeycomb pattern; a few cells on the periphery of the sheet display their long axis; high magnification, SurePath preparation, Papanicolaou stain

with ovulation or the secretory, postovulatory phase of the menstrual cycle [1–3]. The significance of the protrusions has never been firmly established. Usually the cytoplasm is filled with fine, almost transparent mucin or small vacuoles, or may have a larger vacuole resembling a goblet cell, but in some cells the cytoplasm may be dense. Most commonly the cytoplasm stains blue-gray with the Papanicolaou stain. A string of endocervical cells in profile will be aligned in the so-called picket fence or palisade arrangement. If the view is rotated 90°, the cells will appear in a geometric arrangement reminiscent of a honeycomb. In the latter case, varying the microscopic focus will bring either the nuclear pole or the mucin-filled cytoplasmic pole into view (Fig. 3.7). Ciliated endocervical cells are common, especially when the sample has been obtained by vigorous brushing of the upper endocervical canal where ciliated cells are present in increased numbers. A terminal bar anchoring the cilia is often identified (Fig. 3.8).

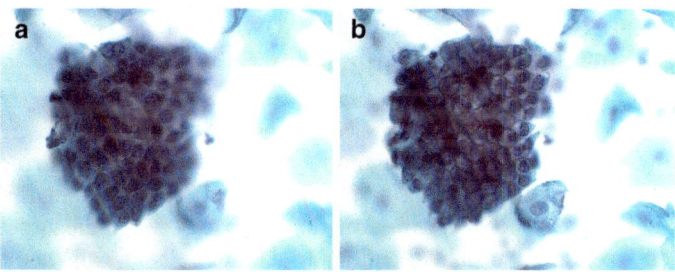

Fig. 3.7 By adjusting the plane of microscopic focus in examining a honeycomb sheet of endocervical cells either the nuclear pole (**a**) or the mucin pole (**b**) can be viewed; both images high magnification, SurePath preparation, Papanicolaou stain

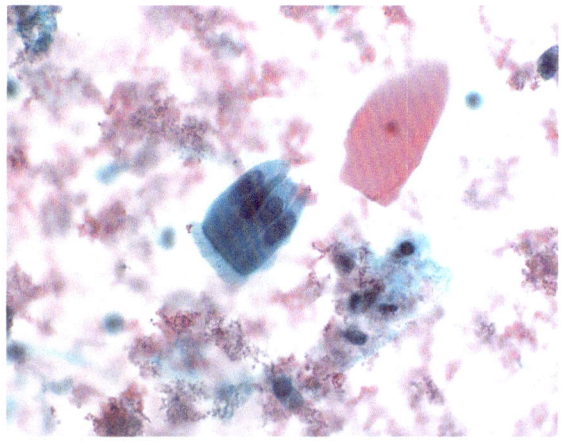

Fig. 3.8 Cilia and the terminal bar of normal endocervical cells; medium magnification, SurePath preparation, Papanicolaou stain

Both the cilia and terminal bar stain either blue or pink with the Papanicolaou stain. The height of the endocervical cell, the opacity of the cytoplasm, and the position of the nucleus have been reported to vary with the phase of the menstrual cycle and the geographic location within the canal [4].

# Histology of the Normal Lower Uterine Segment and Endometrium

On histology sections, the gradual transition of the endocervical mucosa to endometrium in the isthmus or lower uterine segment of the uterus can be appreciated (Fig. 3.9). In this region, the cells become intermediate in size between the larger endocervical and smaller endometrial lining cells, and also show intermediate degrees of pseudostratified architecture.

The cavity of uterine corpus is lined by endometrial mucosa or endometrium, comprises endometrial glands and stroma, both of which undergo cyclic changes during reproductive years. During the first half of the menstrual cycle, the endometrial glands are characterized by mitotic activity in pseudostratified cuboidal to low columnar cells (Fig. 3.10a). The glands advance from straight tubes to tortuous structures with the appearance of subnuclear vacuoles as ovulation at the midpoint of the cycle is approached. The hallmarks of the secretory phase include alignment of the subnuclear vacuoles with eventual secretion into the glandular lumens. Mitotic activity is

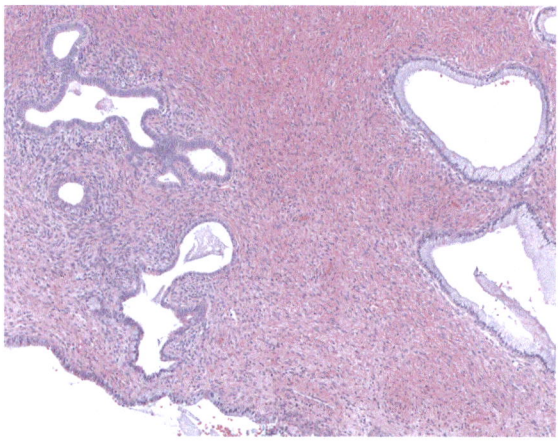

Fig. 3.9 Histologic sections of lower uterine segment with endocervix to the right transitioning to endometrial type stromal and glands to the *left* of the image; low magnification, hematoxylin and eosin stain

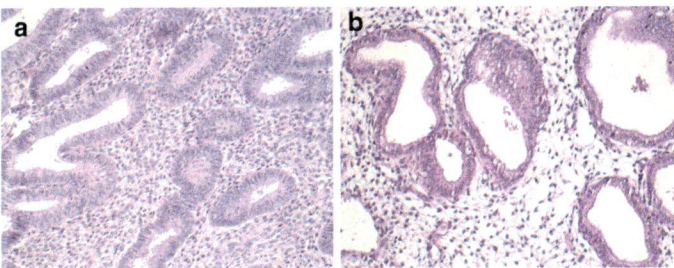

FIG. 3.10 Mitotically active glands of proliferative endometrium with cigar-shaped nuclei staggered around the gland lumen (**a**); dilated, variably vacuolated glands of secretory endometrium (**b**); both images medium magnification, hematoxylin and eosin stain

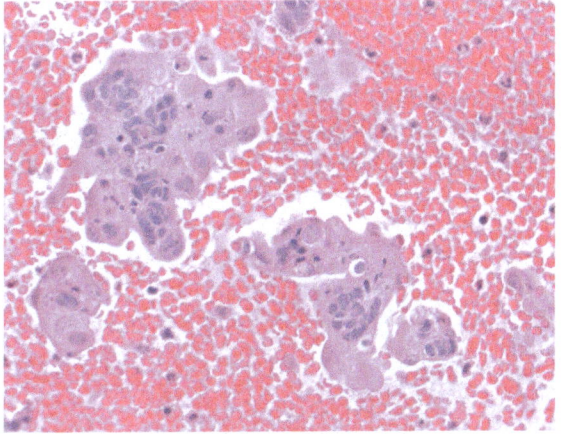

FIG. 3.11 Menstrual endometrium characterized by endometrial gland epithelium surrounding collapsed stroma; medium magnification, hematoxylin and eosin stain

no longer apparent in the endometrial cells of the increasingly serrated glands (Fig. 3.10b). The stroma of the secretory phase shows prominent edematous change followed by prominence of spiral arteries and finally dense pseudo-decidualization with infiltration by inflammatory cells. Late-secretory glands become tightly packed with prominent cytoplasmic vacuoles. If pregnancy does not occur, the endometrial glands and stroma collapse and are shed (Fig. 3.11).

## Cytology of Endometrium

Endometrium shed during the menstrual cycle will appear differently from directly sampled endometrium. During the reproductive years, the endometrium is shed mainly during the first half of the menstrual cycle. During the first days of the cycle, abundant blood, cellular debris, and clusters of endometrial cells will be identified. Larger fragments of shed endometrium will ensue. The typical appearance is that of a three-dimensional sphere of enlarged, often vacuolated endometrial glandular cells with associated apoptotic debris surrounding a central core of tightly compressed, somewhat elongate stromal nuclei (Fig. 3.12). Clusters that comprise only endometrial glandular cells are distinguished from endocervical cells by their generally smaller size, scant cytoplasm, and their three-dimensional arrangement (Fig. 3.13). Some endometrial glandular cells can have prominent cytoplasmic vacuoles best seen on the periphery of the groups. Occasionally, the vacuoles can be filled with polymorphonuclear leukocytes,

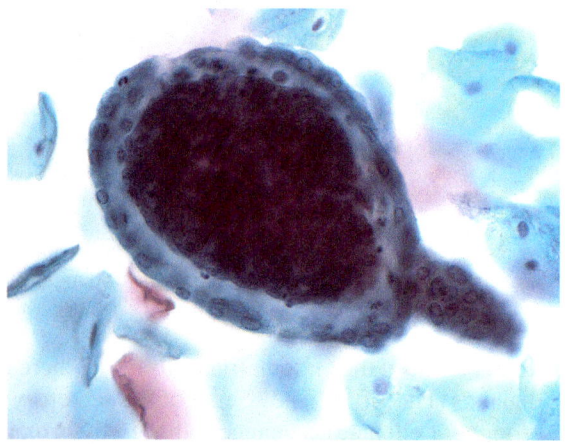

Fig. 3.12 Cytologic appearance of shed endometrium with tightly packed central core of endometrial stromal cells surrounded by uniform benign epithelium, an endometrial wreath; medium magnification, SurePath preparation, Papanicolaou stain

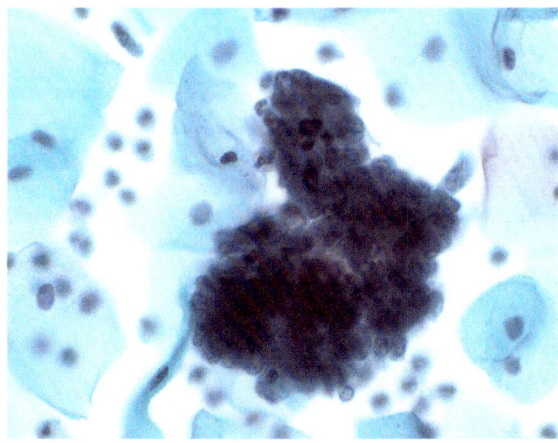

Fig. 3.13 A cluster of shed endometrial cells is more crowded and smaller than benign endocervical cells; high magnification, SurePath preparation, Papanicolaou stain

a finding that is not indicative of a neoplasm, but only a degenerative change within the shed endometrial glandular cells (Fig. 3.14). Fragments of tightly packed endometrial stromal cells with little or no discernible cytoplasm and convoluted small dark nuclei may also be shed (Fig. 3.15a). Single cells resembling small macrophages shed during the initial days of the menstrual cycle were thought to be modified endometrial stromal cells by Papanicolaou who coined the term "exodus" for their abundance (Fig. 3.15b). In fact, it is now accepted that shed superficial stromal cells are indistinguishable from loose clusters of histiocytes [5].

Shed clusters of endometrial cells as well as endocervical cells, often with prominent cytoplasmic vacuoles, nuclear enlargement, and prominent nucleoli, occur regularly in women who use an intrauterine device (IUD) (Fig. 3.16). Their presence is thought to be due to constant irritation of the lining of the corpus and lower uterine segment.

Before the age of 40 years, shed endometrial cells identified on cervical cytology are not reported, regardless of when the cells appear during the menstrual cycle, because the occurrence

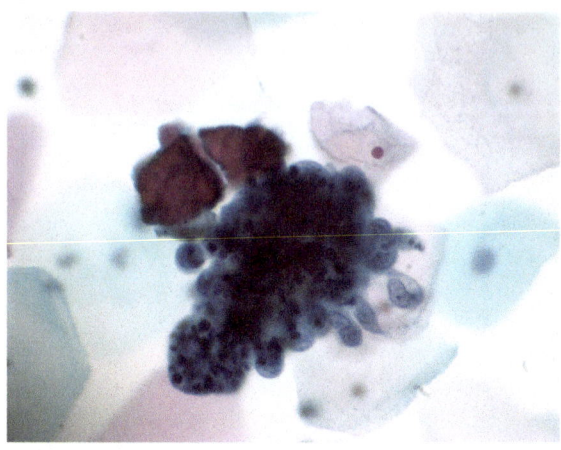

FIG. 3.14 A cluster of shed endometrial cells. Note the cell to the right with vacuolated cytoplasm protruding from the group. This is a typical finding in SurePath preparations Also note the abundance of neutrophils filling the cytoplasm of an adjacent cell, a characteristic of endometrial glandular cells. The amorphous material to the *upper left* of the cell group is degenerated blood; high magnification, SurePath preparation, Papanicolaou stain

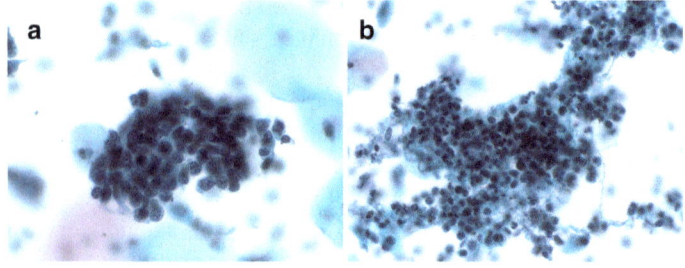

FIG. 3.15 (**a**) A crowded group of small polygonal endometrial stromal cells; high magnification, SurePath preparation, Papanicolaou stain. (**b**) A more loosely cohesive shed group of endometrial cells in a pattern known as "exodus"; medium magnification, SurePath preparation, Papanicolaou stain

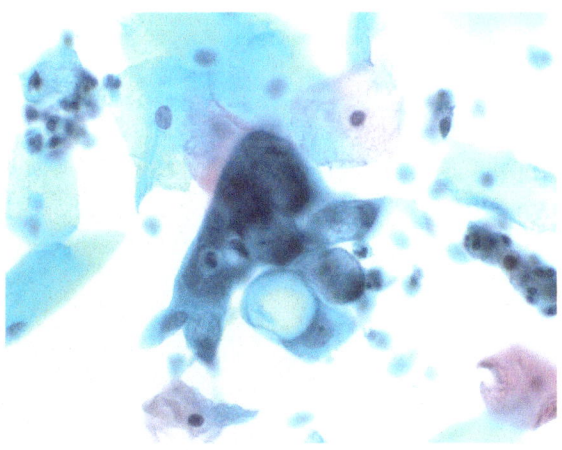

FIG. 3.16 Hypervacuolated glandular cells (endometrial or endocervical) are often identified in women with an intrauterine device in place; high magnification, SurePath preparation, Papanicolaou stain

of associated endometrial pathology in young women is too rare, and the presence of physiologic anovulatory abnormalities too common, to warrant a diagnostic work-up. However, over the age of 40 and especially when a woman is beyond her reproductive years, the presence of shed endometrium may herald endometrial hyperplasia or neoplasia. This risk is relatively low in the first decade after 40, but increases steadily in the following decades. Thus the clinician should be alerted to the presence of shed, albeit benign-appearing endometrium, particularly in the circumstance where it is known that a woman is postmenopausal, or where an accurate menstrual history is not obtained. This result should be accompanied by an explanatory note to alert the clinician to the low but real risk of underlying endometrial pathology [5–7].

The new sampling devices for cervical cytology, especially endocervical brushes and brooms, can commonly obtain directly sampled endometrium from the lower uterine segment [8]. This is particularly true for women who have had excisional procedures of the cervix, such as loop electrosurgical excision procedure (LEEP) or a cone biopsy which results in a shorter distance to the lower uterine segment [9].

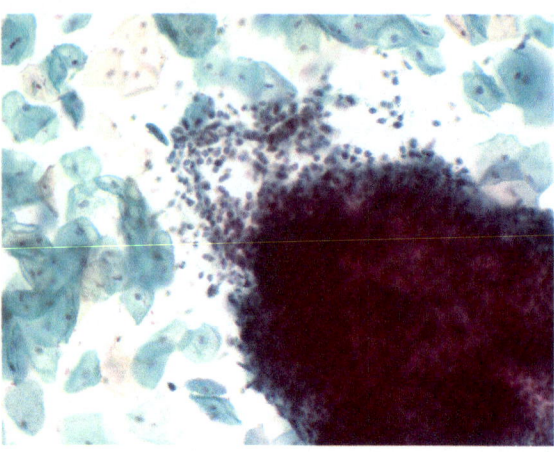

FIG. 3.17  A large fragment of endometrial stroma from which single stromal cells are shed; low magnification, SurePath preparation, Papanicolaou stain

On cytology, direct sampling of the lower uterine segment can be suspected at low power. Large crowded sheets of endometrial stromal cells are found and may cause concern for the presence of a high grade squamous lesion or endocervical glandular neoplasia, but on high power inspection the endometrial stromal cells are much smaller than endocervical glandular cells or squamous cells and show tapered ends generally peeling off from the margins of the groups, a feature which is indicative of their mesenchymal origin (Fig. 3.17). The large stromal fragments will often have embedded tubular glands that stand out at scanning power (Fig. 3.18). Occasionally a tubular gland will be found not in association with stromal fragments and will present in isolation. In such circumstances, attention to detail will usually show adherent stromal cells attached to the basal portions of the endometrial glands, a finding that would not be present typically in neoplastic lesions. Abraded groups of ciliated endocervical cells with attached endometrial type stroma may also be identified in a sample from the lower uterine segment (Fig. 3.19).

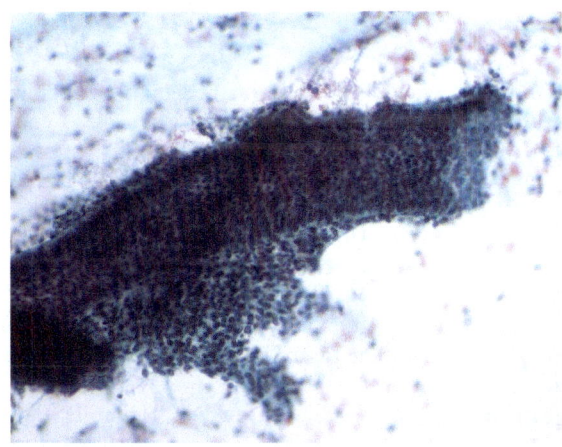

FIG. 3.18 Directly sampled endometrial stroma with an embedded tubular endometrial gland; low magnification, conventional smear, Papanicolaou stain

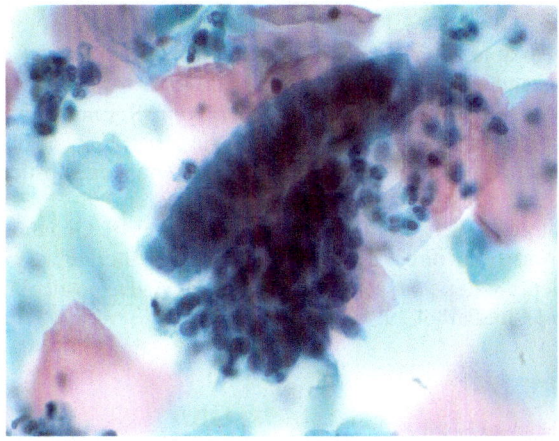

FIG. 3.19 Direct sampling of lower uterine segment: ciliated endocervical cells are attached to cellular endometrial stroma; high magnification, SurePath preparation, Papanicolaou stain

# References

1. McCallum SM. New observations on the significance of nipplelike protrusions in the nuclei of endocervical cells. Acta Cytol. 1988;32(3):331–4.
2. Koizumi JH. Nipplelike protrusions in endocervical and other cells: further observations. Acta Cytol. 1996;40(3):519–28.
3. Zaharopoulos P, Wong J, Wen JW. Nuclear protrusions in cells from cytologic specimens. Mechanisms of formation. Acta Cytol. 1998;42(2):317–29.
4. Affandi MZ, Doctor V, Jhaveri K. The endocervical smear as a simple and quick method for the determination of ovulation. Acta Cytol. 1985;29(4):638–41.
5. Greenspan DL, Cardillo M, Davey DD, Heller DS, Moriarty AT. Endometrial cells in cervical cytology: review of cytological features and clinical assessment. J Low Genit Tract Dis. 2006;10(2):111–22.
6. Aslan DL, Crapanzano JP, Harshan M, Erroll M, Vakil B, Pirog EC. The Bethesda System 2001 recommendation for reporting of benign appearing endometrial cells in Pap tests of women age 40 years and older leads to unwarranted surveillance when followed without clinical qualifiers. Gynecol Oncol. 2007;107(1):86–93.
7. Jones E, Frain BM, Crabtree W. Clinical significance of reporting benign-appearing endometrial cells in Pap tests in women aged 40 years and over. Acta Cytol. 2009;53(1):18–23.
8. de Peralta-Venturino MN, Purslow MJ, Kini SR. Endometrial cells of the "lower uterine segment" (LUS) in cervical smears obtained by endocervical brushings: a source of potential diagnostic pitfall. Diagn Cytopathol. 1995;12(3):263–8; discussion 268–71.
9. Heaton Jr RB, Harris TF, Larson DM, Henry MR. Glandular cells derived from direct sampling of the lower uterine segment in patients status post-cervical cone biopsy. A diagnostic dilemma. Am J Clin Pathol. 1996;106(4):511–6.

# Chapter 4
# Cytology of Endocervical Glandular Neoplasia

## Histology and Cytology of Glandular Lesions of the Cervix: Neoplastic and Equivocal

Malignant and premalignant glandular neoplasms of the cervix have been for the most part well-defined histologically in the literature, although not every entity is accepted by all [1]. The leading authority on cervical neoplasms is the World Health Organization Classification of Tumors [2, 3]. Adenocarcinomas can be purely glandular or associated with a nonglandular component (Table 4.1).

## Adenocarcinoma, Usual Type, Invasive and In Situ

About 80 % of cervical adenocarcinoma is of the usual type, which is made up of medium sized mucin-poor glands with eosinophilic cytoplasm, many mitoses and apoptotic debris [4]. The nuclei are hyperchromatic, more elongate than round and have scattered mitotic figures (Fig. 4.1a). The nuclear cytology is generally of intermediate grade. The cytoplasm is usually more eosinophilic and granular than normal endocervical glands which most often show a frothy texture (Fig. 4.1b).

R.H. Tambouret and D.C. Wilbur, *Glandular Lesions of the Uterine Cervix*, Essentials in Cytopathology 19, DOI 10.1007/978-1-4939-1989-5_4, © Springer Science+Business Media New York 2015

TABLE 4.1 Histologically recognized malignant and premalignant glandular lesions of the cervix

| Adenocarcinoma, usual type, in situ and invasive |
| --- |
| Villoglandular adenocarcinoma |
| Mucinous adenocarcinoma |
| Endometrioid adenocarcinoma |
| Clear cell adenocarcinoma |
| Serous adenocarcinoma |
| Mesonephric adenocarcinoma |
| Adenosquamous carcinoma |

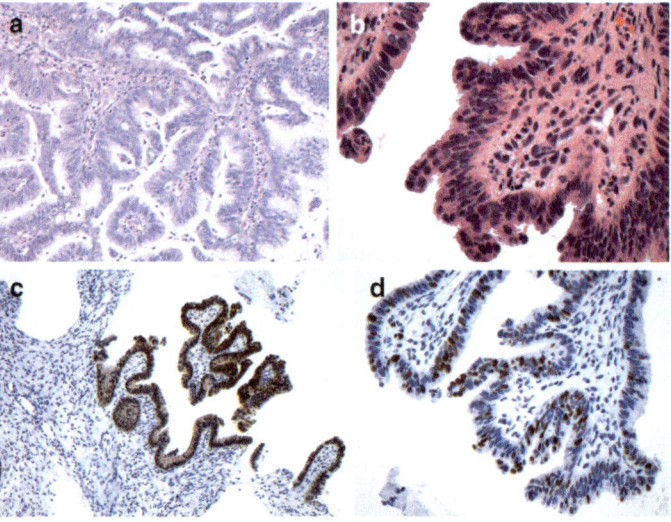

FIG. 4.1 (**a**) Mucin poor glands of the usual type of endocervical adenocarcinoma present in a cribriform pattern. Note the elongate, staggered nuclei within the glands, low power, hematoxylin and eosin stain. (**b**) Hyperchromatic nuclei characteristic of the usual type endocervical adenocarcinoma are apparent, high power, hematoxylin and eosin stain. (**c**) Immunohistochemical staining of the nuclei and cytoplasm of the usual type of endocervical adenocarcinoma for p16 occurs due to the cell cycle dysregulation induced by aberrant activity of high risk HPV, low power. (**d**) In the usual type of endocervical adenocarcinoma many of the tumor cells express Ki67 antigen signifying the active phase of the cell cycle secondary to the effect of high risk HPV as demonstrated by immunohistochemical staining within tumor nuclei, high power

Architecturally, the usual type of endocervical adenocarcinoma can be solid, gland forming, or cribriform. As noted earlier nearly 100 % of the usual type of endocervical adenocarcinomas, invasive and in situ, are positive for hrHPV. Confirmatory tests related to the hrHPV, such as immunohistochemical staining for p16 and Ki67, may be performed on tissue samples, and show typical strong and diffuse "block" positivity and high proliferation indices, respectively (Fig. 4.1c, d). On histology, the features of early invasion may be subtle for several reasons [1]. Tumors may elicit a stromal response, either with stromal density, swirling fibroblastic proliferation, or with chronic inflammation. However, these stromal changes may not always be present and may not be prominent. In addition, adenocarcinoma in situ (AIS) may be intermixed with the invasive component, making their morphologic separation difficult.

In situ forms of the usual type of endocervical adenocarcinoma comprise areas where the normal lobular structure of the endocervical glands is preserved and the normal simple non-stratified epithelium is replaced by a pseudostratified epithelium showing similar cytology to that described above for invasive carcinoma. AIS can be either well differentiated in which the nuclear cytologic changes are minimal, to moderately and poorly differentiated lesions, which show more marked nuclear cytologic atypia.

# The Cytologic Features of the Usual Type of In Situ and Invasive Cervical Adenocarcinoma

## Endocervical Adenocarcinoma In Situ, Usual Type

**Features:**
- Hyperchromatic crowded groups commonly noted initially at low magnification
- Feathering at the periphery of groups
- Rosettes (gland-like formations) within groups

- Cellular disorganization—loss of rigid "honeycombed" structure
- Enlarged nuclei, often elongate
- Coarse chromatin which is generally evenly distributed within the nucleus
- Increased nuclear to cytoplasmic ratio
- Mitoses and apoptotic debris are common

Endocervical AIS is the prototypical endocervical neoplastic lesion which forms the comparator for all discussions of cervical glandular atypia. The cytologic features of endocervical AIS were first described in studies from the mid-1970s [5]. Additional and more detailed descriptions appeared in the 1980s. Prior to TBS 2001, AIS was included only under "Atypical Glandular Cells of Undetermined Significance" (AGUS) because it was not felt to be reliably recognized and reproducible as a discrete category of interpretation. In the intervening time before the publication of the second edition of the Bethesda System (TBS) atlas, the cytologic characterization of AIS had become sufficiently established to be included as a discrete entity. Because cytologists around the world use the TBS atlas as a reference, acceptance of these published criteria for the cytologic diagnosis of AIS has been high and successful application is now more widespread.

The cytologic features of AIS were first described in conventional smears (CS). With the introduction of liquid-based cytology (LBC) preparations in the mid-1990s, subsequent reports described the cytologic features of AIS on LBC along with the differences that had been noted when compared to CS. Although some cytologists, most notably the authors of the second edition of the TBS atlas, felt that the cytologic features of AIS were less readily recognized on LBC because of the three-dimensionality of this specimen type, many studies have concluded that the identification of AIS on LBC samples is also reliable.

The cytologic features of AIS can be subdivided into those that are detectable at low magnification (×10) and those more readily discernible at higher magnifications. Low magnification features are those that are most commonly found on initial

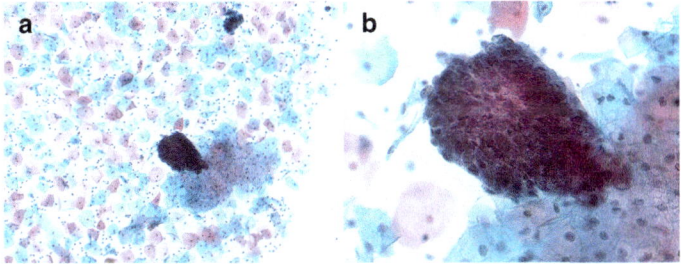

FIG. 4.2 (**a**) A hyperchromatic crowded group (HCG) of cells can be identified at low magnification but to determine the type of cells comprising the group requires higher magnification, SurePath preparation, Papanicolaou stain. (**b**) In this high magnification image the picket fence alignment of the cells on the periphery of the group and the presence of cilia indicates a glandular origin, SurePath preparation, Papanicolaou stain

screening and include the presence of hyperchromatic crowded groups (HCG) of cells. The presence of such groups should always alert the screener to the possibility of a glandular lesion (Fig. 4.2a), and should be carefully examined. At higher magnifications, characteristic architectural features that may suggest an endocervical neoplasia include marked crowding of very dark cells which are irregularly arranged and show nuclear overlap (Fig. 4.2b). With adjustment of the focal plane, the disorganization of the crowded cell groups will be appreciated. As the objective changes plane, the presence of rosettes, abnormal honeycomb formations, and pseudostratification of nuclei can be appreciated. At the margins of the groups, cells and nuclei protrude from the periphery of the crowded cell groups (Fig. 4.3). This is a characteristic feature of AIS which is termed feathering, and may also be a "screening" feature of glandular neoplasia identified at low magnification. In feathering, portions of cytoplasm or protruding nuclei may appear to be falling off the edges of the crowded cell groupings. Feathering is more prominent in conventionally prepared specimens due to the flattening of the groups during the smearing process. The group edges tend

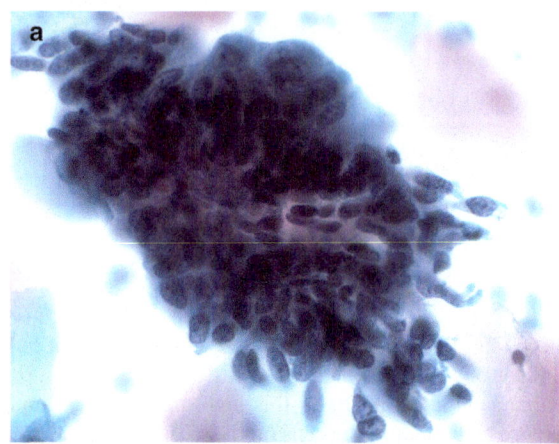

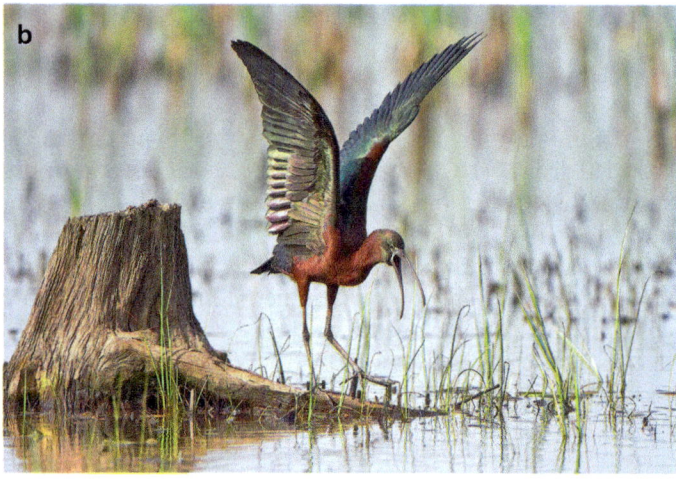

FIG. 4.3  A cell or nucleus protruding from a crowded group of glandular cells is known as feathering (**a**), high power, SurePath preparation, Papanicolaou stain. For comparison an actual bird feather is illustrated (**b**) (Audubon Calendar, reprinted with permission from Dr. Dotty Rosenthal)

to be more blunted in LBC preparations due to the rounding effects of liquid suspension and fixation. In contrast to the crowded glandular groups, single cells or clusters of only 2–3 cells of endocervical AIS are less commonly encountered, but

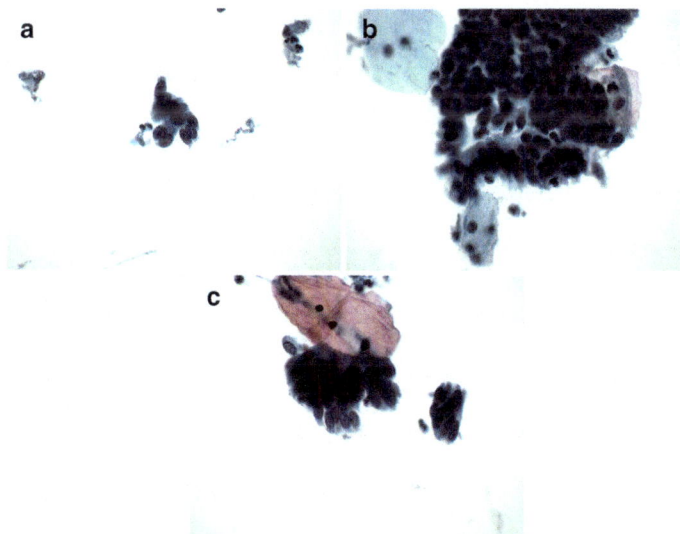

FIG. 4.4 Cells of AIS may be present as single cells or as small groups of abnormal glandular cells (**a**) or in larger groups showing either two-dimensional configuration (**b**) or as pseudostratified strips of cells (**c**). Note the abnormally granular chromatin that is evenly distributed throughout the nuclei in all of these images; all images high power, ThinPrep preparation, Papanicolaou stain

still should be present in most cases and can aid in diagnosis when cells in the hyperchromatic groups cannot be well visualized (Fig. 4.4a, b, c). Glandular lumen or rosette formation, which is indicative of glandular differentiation, may be identified (Fig. 4.5a, b). Pseudostratified strips of columnar cells are commonly present and recapitulate this feature well described in the histology of AIS (Fig. 4.4c).

The nuclei of AIS are enlarged, generally at least twice the area of intermediate squamous cell nuclei (Fig. 4.6a, b). Increased optical density, the so-called hyperchromasia, of the coarsened but evenly distributed chromatin is present. Nuclei may be rounded but often are more elongate than is seen in normal endocervical cells. The nuclear to cytoplasmic ratio is increased. Mitotic figures will often be identified, as well as apoptotic debris, both indicative of high cell turnover

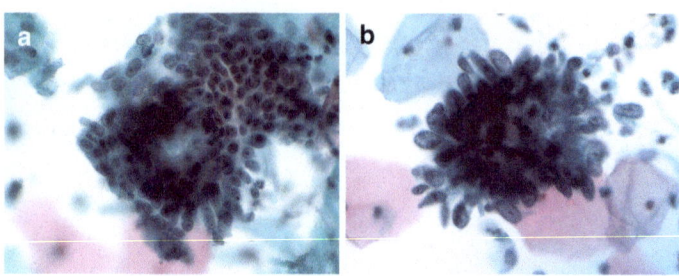

Fig. 4.5 (**a**) A lumen with a clear luminal space present within a cluster of AIS, high power, SurePath preparation, Papanicolaou stain. (**b**) Group of AIS with nuclei oriented toward a central point forming a rosette and demonstrating "feathering," high power, SurePath preparation, Papanicolaou stain

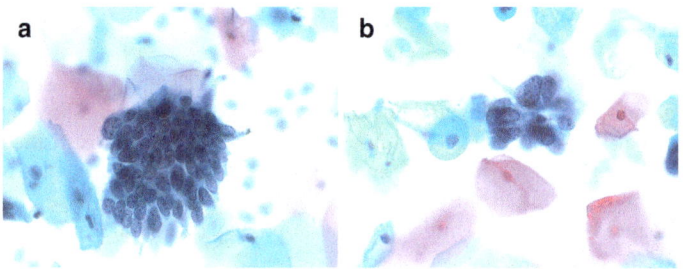

Fig. 4.6 (**a**) A group of enlarged glandular cells with coarse chromatin from a cytology sample of endocervical adenocarcinoma in situ (AIS), high power, SurePath preparation, Papanicolaou stain. (**b**) A deceptively small group of cells of AIS exhibiting coarse chromatin, high power, SurePath preparation, Papanicolaou stain

(Fig. 4.7a, b). As noted in the histology descriptions of the usual type of AIS, most lesions are well differentiated; however, occasional examples will show a more poorly differentiated and therefore more highly atypical nuclear morphology. In such cases, the nuclei can be very large and pleomorphic. In such cases it can be very difficult to distinguish an in situ from an invasive lesion.

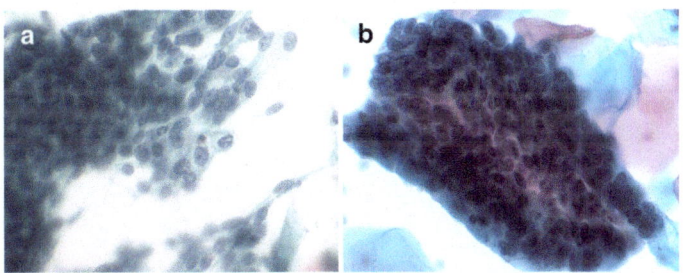

FIG. 4.7 (**a**) A large group of AIS with mitotic figure in a cell on the edge of the group. (**b**) A crowded group of AIS with small fragments of broken down chromatin signifying apoptosis. Both images are high power, SurePath preparation, Papanicolaou stain

In a significant number of cases endocervical AIS is associated with a concurrent squamous lesion, and therefore low- or high grade dysplastic squamous cells may be present in the sample.

At times the crowded cell groups are so densely packed that a distinction between glandular and squamous origin may be a challenge. As noted in Chap. 1, high grade squamous intraepithelial (HSIL) lesions are the most common neoplastic diagnosis in follow-up of an interpretation of atypical glandular cells (AGS), and is the outcome in about 50 % of cases. The cause for this cytologic mimic is the manner of growth of HSIL not only along the surface of the transformation zone, but also the manner of extension into the endocervical crypts. When plucked from the glandular crypts by the sampling device, the HSIL epithelial group maintains a cohesive, bulbous profile, mimicking a HCG of endocervical glandular cells. Clues to the cell of origin are gleaned by examination of the periphery of the HCG where cellular detail is better observed. Columnar shape and delicate mucinous cytoplasm suggest endocervical cells (Fig. 4.8). Flattened, stacked cells suggest a squamous origin (Fig. 4.9). A swirling or spindled cell arrangement deep in the HCG may also suggest squamous differentiation. The cells of HSIL are notorious for growing into and filling native endocervical glands. This HSIL growth

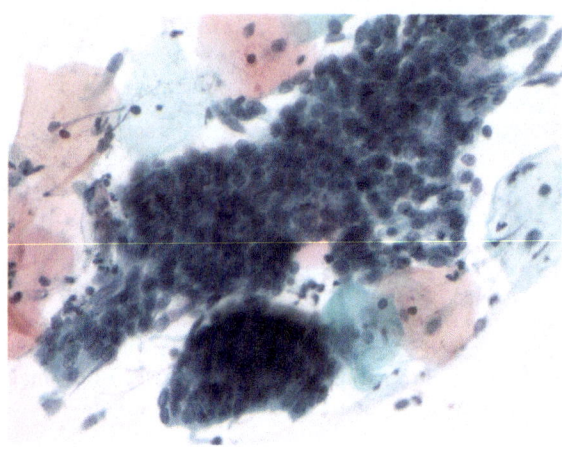

Fig. 4.8 In examining a HCG of cells one should examine the periphery of the group to appreciate the columnar shape of the cell and the mucinous cytoplasm; medium power, SurePath preparation, Papanicolaou stain

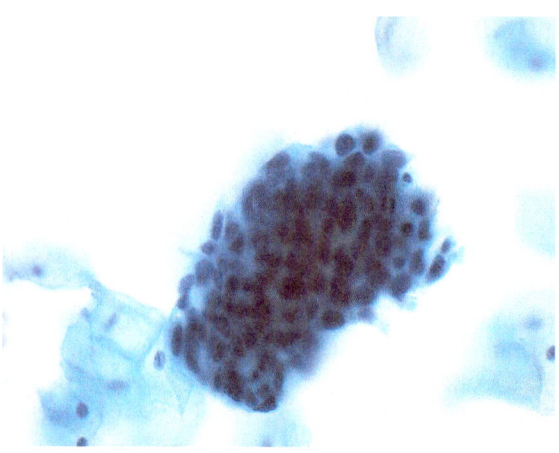

Fig. 4.9 Squamous cells in a crowded hyperchromatic squamous group will have a more flattened or polygonal shape; note mitotic figures; high power, SurePath preparation, Papanicolaou stain

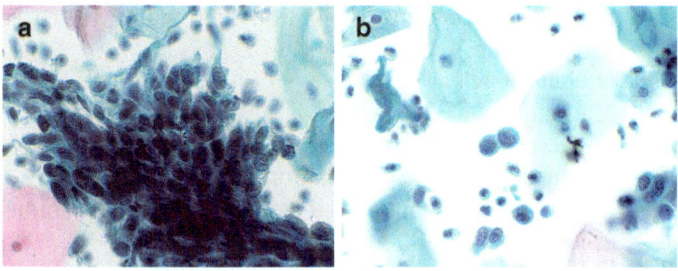

Fɪɢ. 4.10 Cells of high grade squamous intraepithelial lesions (HSIL) often crowd together mimicking a glandular lesion (**a**) but elsewhere on the cytology slide single cells of HSIL will be identified (**b**); both images high power, SurePath preparation, Papanicolaou stain

pattern often will produce crowded groups on cytology that can mimic the groups associated with true glandular lesions (Fig. 4.10a). An important clue to the squamous nature of the lesion will be the presence of single HSIL cells in the background of the slide, which is almost universally noted in specimens found to be derived from squamous mimics of AIS (Fig. 4.10b).

The background of the AIS sample is usually clean, devoid of any necrotic debris or tumor diathesis, indicative of the non-invasive nature of this process. However, occasional cases of AIS can show a prominent inflammatory background pattern.

## *Invasive Endocervical Adenocarcinoma, Usual Type*

**Features:**
- Abundant abnormal columnar cells
- Single cells and crowded groups
- Groups with rosettes, pseudostratification, feathering
- Nuclear enlargement >2–3× intermediate squamous cell nucleus
- Coarsely granular chromatin

- Irregular chromatin distribution (chromatin heterogeneity/clearing)
- Irregular nuclear membrane
- Macronucleoli
- Mitoses, apoptotic debris
- Background of necrosis (tumor diathesis)
- Abnormal squamous cells if associated with a squamous lesion

The authors of the second edition of the Bethesda System have provided criteria for the diagnosis of endocervical adenocarcinoma. An abundance of abnormal cells that are usually columnar in configuration are present in combinations with single cells, flat sheets, and three-dimensional groups of abnormal cells. Direct sampling of lesions accounts for this abundance of cells and also for the two-dimensional architecture. These features can aid in the discrimination from endometrial adenocarcinoma cases, as the latter will comprise fewer cells which are predominantly arranged as three-dimensional tight clusters, indicative of exfoliation and travel in the endocervical mucus. Architectural features of invasive lesions can be similar to AIS, particularly in the well-differentiated variants, and included rosette formation, peripheral drop off of cells from cell groups/feathering, and nuclear pseudostratification. These features are less prominent as the tumors become more poorly differentiated. The nuclei of the abnormal columnar cells are enlarged to at least 2–3 times that of the nucleus of an intermediate squamous cell and may show considerable variation in size and shape. Irregularly distributed chromatin, parachromatin clearing, and nuclear membrane irregularities are characteristic. The malignant nuclei frequently contain macronucleoli. These features can be very useful in the discrimination of well-differentiated invasive lesions from cases of AIS. Mitoses are usually easily identified and cell groups almost always harbor apoptotic debris. The cells have finely vacuolated to granular eosinophilic cytoplasm. Necrosis or tumor diathesis is commonly identified, either as a film in the background of conventional smears or as granular material hugging the malignant cell groups, and a prominent infiltration of inflammatory cells is noted in the background and can sometimes permeate the cell groupings. If a squamous lesion accompanies the adenocarcinoma, abnormal squamous cells will also be identified.

As noted above, considerable overlap of the architectural cytologic criteria exists between AIS and invasive ECA. The principle differences are the presence of tumor necrosis or diathesis in the background in invasive lesions, and the more pronounced degree of nuclear abnormalities in invasive ECA, particularly the uneven nature of the heterochromatin distribution and the presence of chromatin clearing (Fig. 4.11). Careful evaluation of all abnormal glandular groups in a given sample must be performed because AIS is often present alongside invasive ECA and in such circumstances criteria indicative of both lesions will be present in the cytology sample.

As in AIS, large syncytial groups of invasive ECA are usually present in the cytology sample because of direct sampling and usually pose considerable difficulty in interpretation due to the obscuring effect of the cell crowding. Often only the cells on the periphery of the crowded groups are sufficiently visible for adequate analysis (Fig. 4.12).

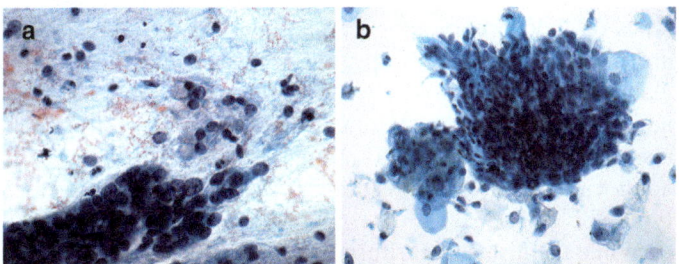

FIG. 4.11 (**a**) Invasive endocervical adenocarcinoma is suspected when a film of necrotic material is present in the background of the cytology sample; low power, conventional smear, Papanicolaou stain. (**b**) On a liquid-based preparation the necrotic debris (tumor diathesis) clings to the malignant glandular groups; medium power, SurePath preparation, Papanicolaou stain

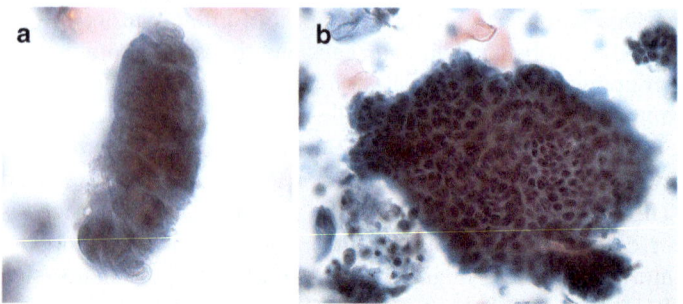

F_IG. 4.12 Cells of well-differentiated adenocarcinoma may be viewed either with the long axis of the cell in profile (**a**) or as if looking down on to the irregular honeycomb pattern (**b**); both images, medium power, SurePath preparation, Papanicolaou stain

# Other Variants of Endocervical Adenocarcinoma: Histologic and Cytologic Presentation

According to the most recent version of the WHO classification, in addition to the most common usual type, seven additional types of endocervical adenocarcinoma, with several variants, are recognized histologically. These include mucinous, villoglandular, endometrioid, clear cell, serous, mesonephric, and adenosquamous types. Minimal deviation adenocarcinoma, also known as adenoma malignum, and intestinal-type adenocarcinoma are considered variants of the mucinous type (Table 4.1).

While the histologic criteria for the different types of invasive endocervical adenocarcinoma (ECA) are well delineated, these distinctions are not as well defined on cytology specimens. The following section will highlight the important features of each tumor type and illustrate, where appropriate, the recognized cytologic features that can be of use in defining these entities in Papanicolaou specimens.

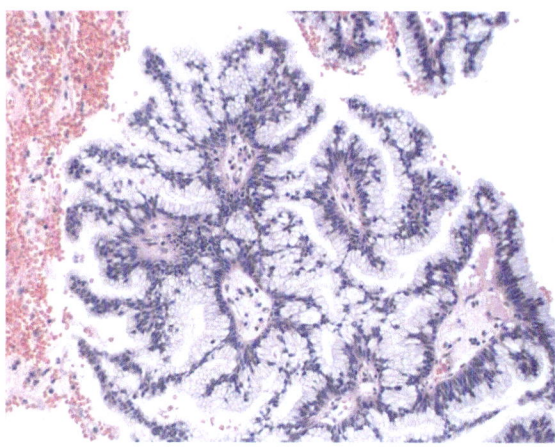

Fig. 4.13 Abundant cytoplasmic mucin is the key feature of mucinous adenocarcinoma of the endocervix, low power, hematoxylin and eosin stain

## Mucinous Type

This tumor is characterized by variably abundant cytoplasmic mucin that is highlighted by mucicarmine stains. Four varieties of this tumor are encountered: gastric-type with prominent apical mucin, intestinal-type with goblet cells, signet ring cell-type and mucinous adenocarcinoma, not otherwise specified, that shares similar histogenesis but which cannot be further classified as to any specific type (Fig. 4.13).

Gastric-type mucinous adenocarcinoma includes the very well-differentiated minimal deviation adenocarcinoma (adenoma malignum). This uncommon tumor makes up less than 5 % of cervical adenocarcinomas in most populations; however, in Japanese populations it has been shown to represent as many as 25 % of cervical adenocarcinoma. Gastric-type adenocarcinoma is most often not associated with high risk HPV and hence HPV testing in follow-up of an "atypical glandular cell" interpretation will not be helpful for the identification of this type of malignancy. This tumor has a distinct association with Peutz-Jeghers syndrome and mutations

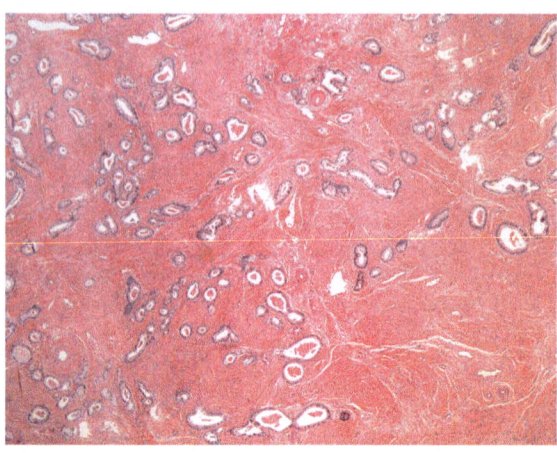

FIG. 4.14 Well-differentiated glands of minimal deviation adenocarcinoma of the cervix are seen invading deeply into the wall of the
cervix, low power, hematoxylin and eosin stain

in a gene for serine threonine kinase (LKB1 or STK11) on
chromosome 19 [6–8].

The original description of minimal deviation adenocarcinoma referred to a very well-differentiated adenocarcinoma
that cytologically resembled normal endocervical glands [9].
The architectural arrangement of the glands is the key to diagnosis with glands being present deep in the cervical wall
(greater than 7 mm) and adjacent to large vessel where normal
endocervical glands would not be present (Fig. 4.14). Often
there is no stromal reaction to the invasive tumor [9].

The cytologic and architectural features of MDACA are
notoriously subtle and may not permit reliable and reproducible recognition in cytologic specimens if a component of less
well-differentiated adenocarcinoma is absent [10]. Notably,
nuclear pleomorphism can be subtle and not present in all
tumor cells; mitotic activity is absent or variable in number
[10, 11] (Fig. 4.15). An abnormal golden yellow hue of intracytoplasmic mucin with the Papanicolaou stain has been
associated with the presence of intestinal types of mucin in
some cases of MDACA [12, 13] (Fig. 4.16). What may raise an

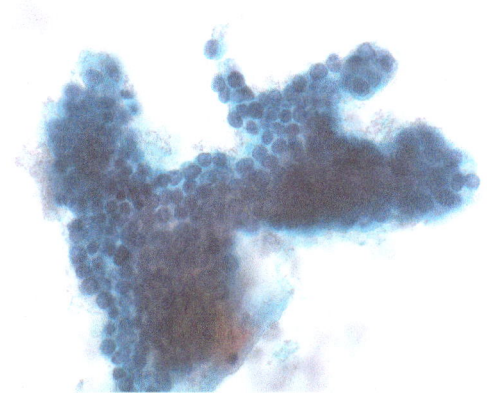

FIG. 4.15 Well-differentiated minimal deviation adenocarcinoma can be very challenging to recognize due to the uniformity of the malignant cells; medium power, SurePath preparation, Papanicolaou stain

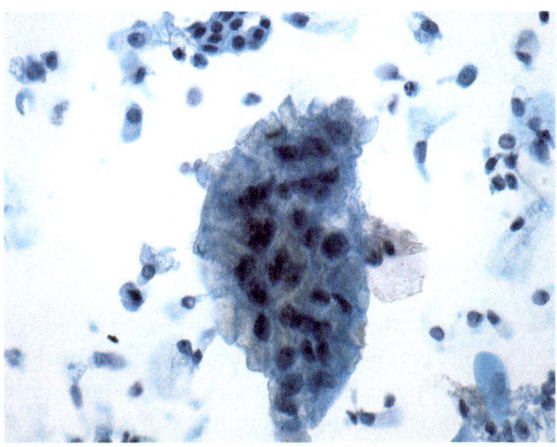

FIG. 4.16 *Golden yellow* intracytoplasmic mucin is found in minimal deviation adenocarcinoma of the endocervix along with disorganized honeycomb pattern, high power, SurePath, Papanicolaou stain

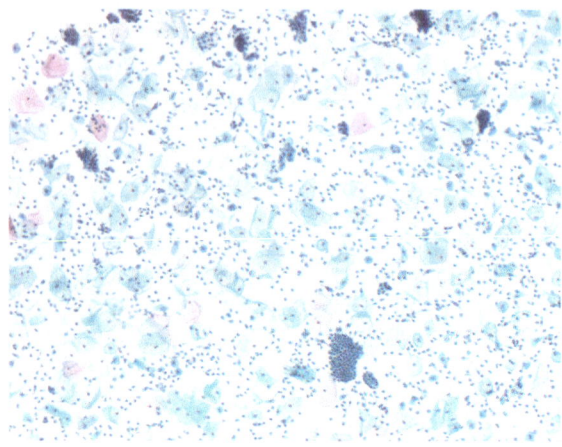

FIG. 4.17  One clue to the presence of very well-differentiated AIS or endocervical adenocarcinoma is the identification of an abnormally large quantity of glandular groups at low magnification; low power, SurePath preparation, Papanicolaou stain

initial screening concern in cases of mucinous adenocarcinoma is the presence of an abnormally high number of endocervical-type glandular cells in the specimen with some mild and variable nuclear enlargement [10], architectural disorganization, and the presence of abundant frothy mucus in the majority of cells, many of which have a "goblet cell configuration" (Fig. 4.17).

## Villoglandular Type

Some cervical adenocarcinomas may have a minor or pronounced villous component, but when the bulk of the tumor exhibits an exophytic papillary architecture and only mild cytologic atypia is present, the tumor can be designated as villoglandular adenocarcinoma (Fig. 4.18). This is an important subcategory because it tends to arise in a younger population and because it often shows only minimal superficial invasion; therefore, the tumor is amenable to conservative

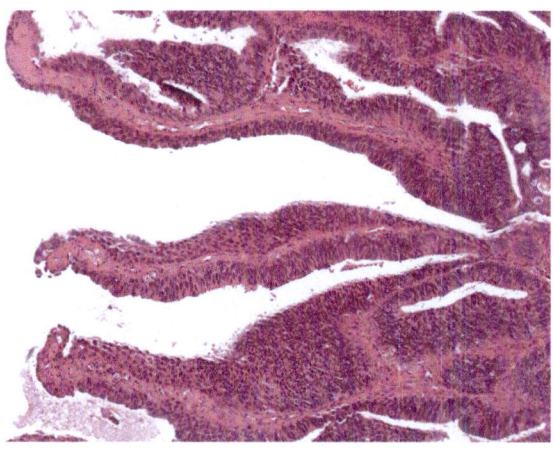

FIG. 4.18 Long slender papillae are features of villoglandular adeno-carcinoma of the cervix, low power, hematoxylin and eosin stain

excision, particularly where maintenance of childbearing is an important consideration.

The cytologic features of villoglandular adenocarcinoma will be similar to the usual type of cervical adenocarcinoma with the caveat that they will always exhibit well-differentiated nuclear features; hence, they will very often resemble cases of AIS. Occasionally architectural structures recapitulating the villous nature of the tumor will be present intact in the specimens.

## Endometrioid Type

The endometrioid type is generally considered to represent no more than 5 % of all cervical adenocarcinomas [14, 15]. This tumor resembles endometrioid adenocarcinoma arising in the uterine corpus and is composed of tubular glands, often with ciliated columnar cells with little or no mucin (Fig. 4.19). The fact that endometrioid carcinomas have a high rate of HPV positivity suggests that endometrioid is an overlapping

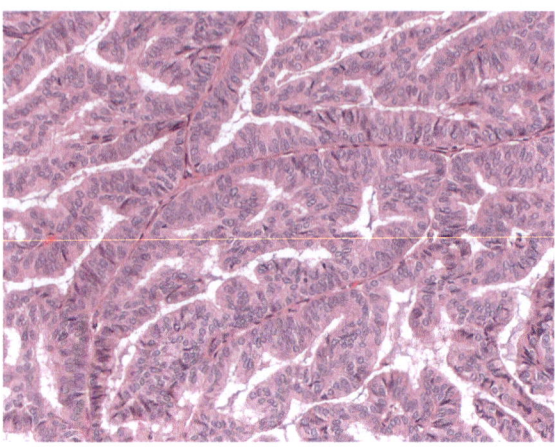

Fig. 4.19  Cervical biopsy with crowded mucin-poor glands of endo-metrioid adenocarcinoma of the cervix, medium power, hematoxylin and eosin stain

morphologic variant of the usual type, since tumors arising from the endometrium will be HPV negative.

From the cytologic standpoint, the most important feature of endometrioid types of neoplasms is the small size of the nuclei compared to those of the usual type, and the densely packed nature of the groups in which they present. The endo-metrioid type of AIS is important because it has been fre-quently misinterpreted as normal high endocervical or lower uterine segment (LUS) sampling [16, 17]. In endometrioid type of AIS, the relatively small tightly packed cells appear as crowded groups (Fig. 4.20). Although the chromatin is hyper-chromatic and coarse, the nuclei are small and relatively uniform. Both mitoses and nuclear/cytoplasmic feathering may be seen at the periphery of the cell groups. Unlike directly sampled endometrial cells from the LUS, endometrial stromal cells will not be attached to the surfaces of the tightly packed glandular cells in endometrioid AIS, and the presence of pure endometrial stromal groups will not be present in the background.

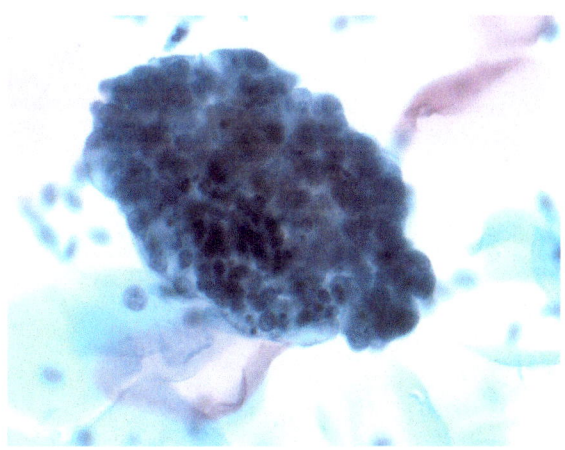

Fig. 4.20 An example of endometrioid type of AIS presents as a tight cluster of glandular cells with enlarged, dark nuclei and prominent cytoplasmic vacuoles most evident at the periphery of the group; high power, SurePath preparation, Papanicolaou stain

## Clear Cell Type

Prior to the administration of diethylstilbestrol (DES) during pregnancy, clear cell adenocarcinoma was uncommon. For at least three decades clear cell carcinoma occurred at an increased frequency in women exposed to DES in utero and although DES is no longer prescribed, clear cell carcinoma continues to be seen. The tumor is characterized by tubulocystic, papillary, or solid architectural patterns with cells having abundant clear to scant glycogen rich cytoplasm, and high grade nuclear atypia (Fig. 4.21).

## Serous Type

Although the tumor may rarely be primary, when serous adenocarcinoma is found in the cervix, the tumor is more likely to have arisen elsewhere in the female genital tract. Serous adenocarcinoma shares the same morphology as

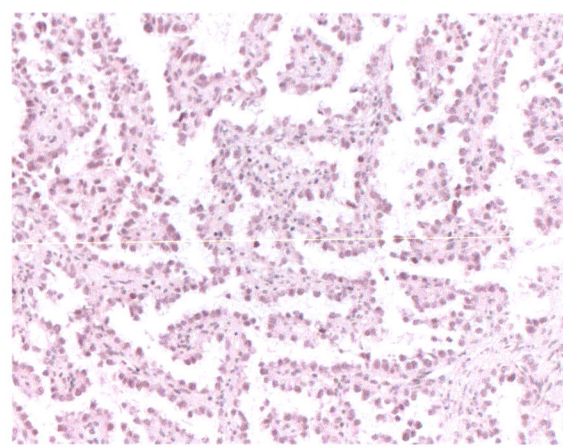

Fig. 4.21 Tubular glands of clear cell carcinoma of the cervix; the tumor nuclei are hyperchromatic contrasting with the delicate, optically clear cytoplasm, medium power, hematoxylin and eosin stain

serous carcinomas found in the ovary, fallopian tube, and endometrium and consists of high grade tumor cells forming crowded papillae which can be compressed to form slit-like spaces (Fig. 4.22).

The cytologic features of clear cell and serous carcinomas are overlapping and consist of high grade nuclear features often showing prominent hobnail group configurations and eosinophilic or vacuolated cytoplasm. These tumors are not difficult to recognize as malignant, but their presence in a cytologic specimen more commonly raises the possibility of a metastasis as opposed to a primary cervical neoplasm.

## Mesonephric Type

Mesonephric adenocarcinoma, the rarest subtype of cervical adenocarcinoma, is composed of densely packed small, round glands containing dense, eosinophilic material within the gland lumens, mimicking the appearance of mesonephric remnants

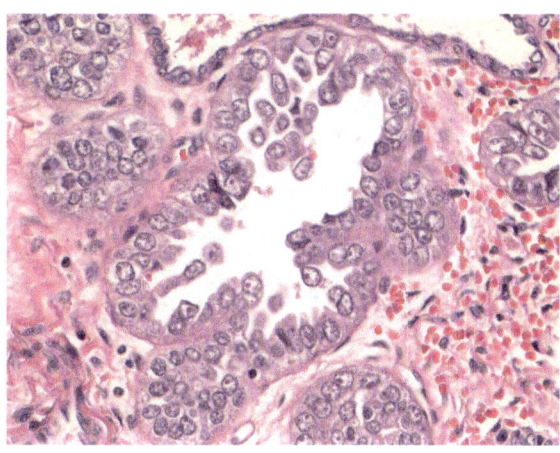

FIG. 4.22 The glands of serous carcinoma are lined by cells with nuclei protruding into the gland lumen creating an irregular lumen contour, medium power, hematoxylin and eosin stain

which can be found as a benign incidental finding in the outer lateral wall of the cervix.

Mesonephric tumors have not been described in the cytology literature, but based on their histologic appearance, they would most closely resemble the usual or endometrioid types. The presence of dense colloid-like material within a gland structure might suggest the presence of mesonephric differentiation.

## Adenosquamous Type

The WHO defines this tumor as one that can be recognized without the use of special stains. The adenocarcinoma component is most often of the usual type, although mucinous, clear cell, or endometrioid may occur (Fig. 4.23). Cytologic features would therefore be as noted above for the glandular component, with a second component showing the typical features of squamous differentiation.

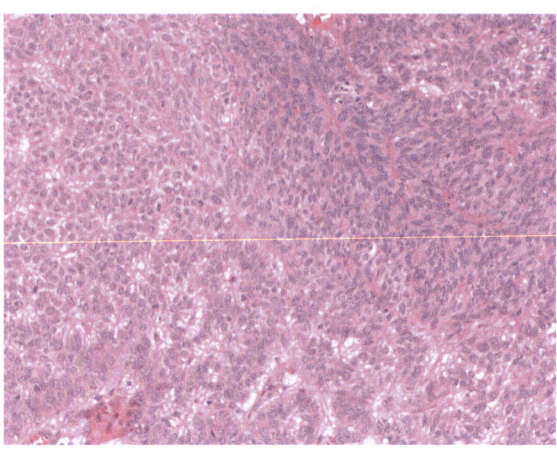

FIG. 4.23 Adenosquamous carcinoma of the endocervix: gland forming tumor is present to the *left* of the image while the more solid tumor to the right suggests squamous differentiation, low power, hematoxylin and eosin stain

## Endocervical Gland Dysplasia and Atypical Endocervical Cells

Unlike cervical squamous epithelium, the cytologic features of precursor or dysplastic glandular lesions of degrees less than AIS have not been well defined, much less graded as to severity. Although the British have adopted the histologic terminology of "cervical glandular intraepithelial neoplasia" (CGIN), controversy surrounds this designation. CGIN is divided into low grade CGIN or glandular dysplasia and high grade CGIN or AIS. Unfortunately low grade CGIN is a poorly reproducible designation [1]. In histologic preparations, the criteria for low grade CGIN include mild nuclear atypia with hyperchromasia and occasional mitotic figures and apoptotic debris. However, according to the revised British Society for Clinical Cytology (BSCC) terminology for abnormal cervical cytology, only high grade CGIN is defined cytologically with criteria completely analogous to those noted above for AIS [18]. The 2001 Bethesda System terminology

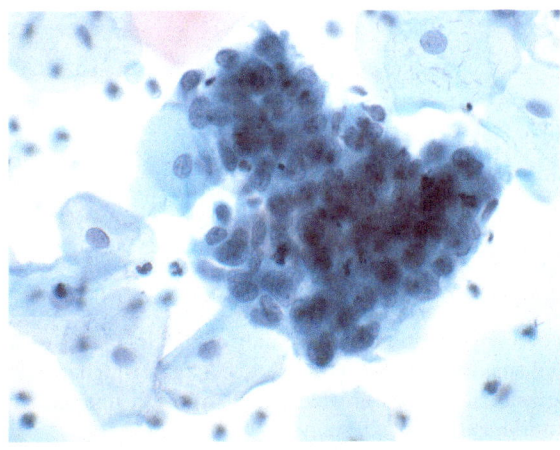

FIG. 4.24 Mitotic activity in endocervical adenocarcinoma; high power, SurePath preparation, Papanicolaou stain

did recognize changes to endocervical glandular cells that did not meet the criteria for AIS but that were sufficiently worrisome to require reporting, and adopted the term "atypical glandular cells—endocervical (AEC)" to reflect the uncertainty associated with these equivocal cytologic features The designation "AEC not otherwise specified" applies when only some but not all of the features of AIS or ECA are present, or the features present are qualitatively insufficient to instill confidence in their application. These features may include nuclear enlargement, degrees of hyperchromasia, nucleoli formation, size variability, cell crowding and nuclear overlap, incomplete rosette formation, and partial pseudostratification. Mitotic figures may be found but should not be numerous, and apoptotic breakdown fragments should not be prominent (Fig. 4.24).

The category of "AEC, favor neoplastic" is used when more pronounced or more numerous abnormalities are present in the endocervical cells, which may include the architectural features of rosettes, feathering, pseudostratified strips, and intermediate numbers of mitoses, but of insufficient extent to allow confidence in an outright interpretation (Fig. 4.25).

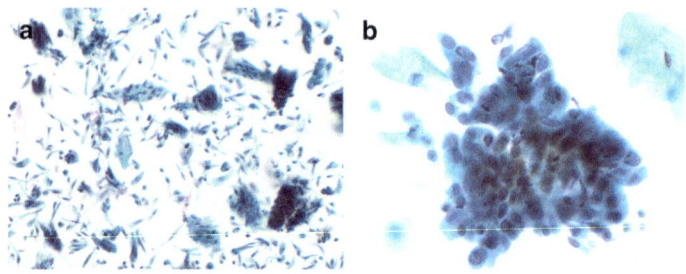

FIG. 4.25  Atypical endocervical cells, favor neoplasia: low magnification of a sample composed almost only of glandular cells with single cells and small fan-shaped groups of cells (**a**); at higher magnification occasional mitoses are identified (**b**); both images, SurePath preparation, Papanicolaou stain

Because AEC is considered an equivocal categorization, the differential diagnosis will include a variety of benign entities, such as reparative changes, endocervical polyps, changes secondary to the presence of an intrauterine device, tubal metaplasia, sampling of the LUS, and pregnancy-related changes (these entities are discussed in greater detail in Chap. 5). Atypical repair at the transformation zone of the cervix can be cause for alarm, most commonly mimicking an invasive lesion because of the presence of tissue damage leading to diathesis patterns in the background and the presence of highly atypical nuclei. HSIL involving glands will often be called AEC on cytology due to the crowded, three-dimensional, hyperchromatic groups, especially on LBC samples.

The prevalence of the designation of a cervical cytology samples as containing AEC and AGC in general should be low, generally far less than 1 % in most studies. This low prevalence is in contrast to the high prevalence of ASC-US interpretations, the latter constituting as much as 5 % in a screening population [19]. However, the rate of significant lesions following an interpretation of AEC is much higher than following an interpretation of ASC-US, and hence the much more aggressive management that is mandated for these lesions. Outcome studies of histologic findings following the cytologic diagnosis of AGC are discussed in Chap. 2. When an interpretation of

AEC is being entertained by the cytologist, every attempt should be made to obtain all available information to help in arriving at as precise a conclusion as possible. This work-up should include obtaining all relevant clinical information, particularly from direct communication with the clinician as often additional relevant information not available in the patient record may be obtained.

## References

1. McCluggage WG. New developments in endocervical glandular lesions. Histopathology. 2013;62(1):138–60.
2. Wells M, Ostor AG, Crum CP, Franceschi S, Tommasino M, Nesland JM, et al. Tumors of the uterine cervix: epithelial tumors. In: Tavassoli FA, Deville P, editors. Pathology and genetics of tumors of the breast and female genital organs. Lyon: IARC; 2003. p. 262–79.
3. Kurman RJ, Carcangiu M-L, Herrington CS, Young RH. WHO classification of tumours of female reproductive organs. Lyon: IARC; 2014.
4. Young RH, Clement PB. Endocervical adenocarcinoma and its variants: their morphology and differential diagnosis. Histopathology. 2002;41(3):185–207.
5. Krumins I, Young Q, Pacey F, Bousfield L, Mulhearn L. The cytologic diagnosis of adenocarcinoma in situ of the cervix uteri. Acta Cytol. 1977;21(2):320–9.
6. Jenne DE, Reimann H, Nezu J, Friedel W, Loff S, Jeschke R, et al. Peutz-Jeghers syndrome is caused by mutations in a novel serine threonine kinase. Nat Genet. 1998;18(1):38–43.
7. Hemminki A. The molecular basis and clinical aspects of Peutz-Jeghers syndrome. Cell Mol Life Sci. 1999;55(5):735–50.
8. Mikami Y, McCluggage WG. Endocervical glandular lesions exhibiting gastric differentiation: an emerging spectrum of benign, premalignant, and malignant lesions. Adv Anat Pathol. 2013;20(4):227–37.
9. Silverberg SG, Hurt WG. Minimal deviation adenocarcinoma ("adenoma malignum") of the cervix: a reappraisal. Am J Obstet Gynecol. 1975;121(7):971–5.
10. Granter SR, Lee KR. Cytologic findings in minimal deviation adenocarcinoma (adenoma malignum) of the cervix. A report of seven cases. Am J Clin Pathol. 1996;105(3):327–33.

11. Szyfelbein WM, Young RH, Scully RE. Adenoma malignum of the cervix. Cytologic findings. Acta Cytol. 1984;28(6):691–8.
12. Ishii K, Katsuyama T, Ota H, Watanabe T, Matsuyama I, Tsuchiya S, et al. Cytologic and cytochemical features of adenoma malignum of the uterine cervix. Cancer. 1999;87(5):245–53.
13. Hata S, Mikami Y, Manabe T. Diagnostic significance of endocervical glandular cells with "golden-yellow" mucin on pap smear. Diagn Cytopathol. 2002;27(2):80–4.
14. Zaino RJ. The fruits of our labors: distinguishing endometrial from endocervical adenocarcinoma. Int J Gynecol Pathol. 2002; 21(1):1–3.
15. Schorge JO, Lee KR, Lee SJ, Flynn CE, Goodman A, Sheets EE. Early cervical adenocarcinoma: selection criteria for radical surgery. Obstet Gynecol. 1999;94(3):386–90.
16. Lee KR, Minter LJ, Granter SR. Papanicolaou smear sensitivity for adenocarcinoma in situ of the cervix. A study of 34 cases. Am J Clin Pathol. 1997;107(1):30–5.
17. Lee KR, Genest DR, Minter LJ, Granter SR, Cibas ES. Adenocarcinoma in situ in cervical smears with a small cell (endometrioid) pattern: distinction from cells directly sampled from the upper endocervical canal or lower segment of the endometrium. Am J Clin Pathol. 1998;109(6):738–42.
18. Denton KJ, Herbert A, Turnbull LS, Waddell C, Desai MS, Rana DN, et al. The revised BSCC terminology for abnormal cervical cytology. Cytopathology. 2008;19(3):137–57.
19. Chhieng DC, Cangiarella JF. Atypical glandular cells. Clin Lab Med. 2003;23(3):633–57.

# Chapter 5
## Cytologic Mimics of Endocervical Glandular Neoplasia

Diagnosis of preneoplastic and neoplastic glandular lesions of the lower genital tract is confounded by the presence of a variety of other cellular processes. When confronted with a potential glandular lesion on cervical cytology, the cytologist should give consideration to and exclude the following mimics of neoplasia.

## Histology of Benign Glandular Lesions of the Cervix

A variety of benign changes can occur in the endocervix which enter into the differential diagnosis when a glandular lesion is suspected on cervical cytology. Before delving into the cytology, a general understanding of the histology of benign lesions is helpful (Table 5.1) [1].

## Histology of Metaplasias and Ectopias

Tubal and tubo-endometrioid metaplasia (TEM) refers to replacement of endocervical epithelial cells by ciliated cells, slender non-ciliated "intercalated" cells with apical snouts,

R.H. Tambouret and D.C. Wilbur, *Glandular Lesions of the Uterine Cervix*, Essentials in Cytopathology 19, DOI 10.1007/978-1-4939-1989-5_5, © Springer Science+Business Media New York 2015

TABLE 5.1  Histologically recognized benign changes of the endocervix

Tubal/tubo-endometrioid metaplasia
Endometriosis
Oxyphil metaplasia
Prostatic tissue metaplasia
Endocervical gland hyperplasia
Mesonephric gland hyperplasia
Reactive atypia of endocervical glands
Viral infection of endocervical gland epithelium
Pregnancy-related changes
Endocervical polyps

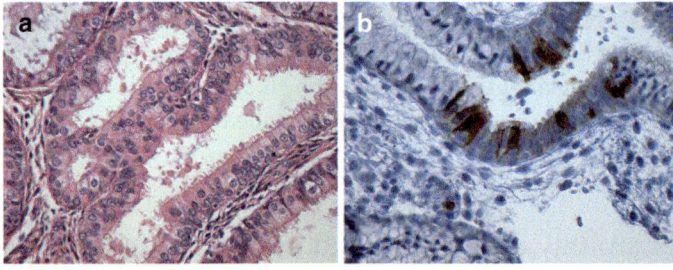

FIG. 5.1  (**a**) Delicate cilia cover the luminal surface of benign endo-cervical glands in tubal metaplasia; medium power, hematoxylin and eosin stain; (**b**) immunohistochemical staining for p16 is positive in isolated cells of tubal metaplasia unlike the diffuse staining pattern seen in the usual type of endocervical adenocarcinoma; medium power, hematoxylin and eosin stain

and the mucinous "peg" cells similar to those of the fallopian tube or endometrial glands [2, 3]. This type of metaplasia is very common in the upper portions of the endocervical canal, particularly in the late childbearing age group (Fig. 5.1).

Superficial cervical endometriosis is recognized by the presence of endometrial glands accompanied by endometrial stroma. Endometriosis is often present just below the surface of the cervical squamous epithelium and may erode through the surface to be sampled in the taking of a Pap test (Fig. 5.2).

Oxyphil metaplasia of endocervical glands results in glands lined by a single layer of columnar cells with dense,

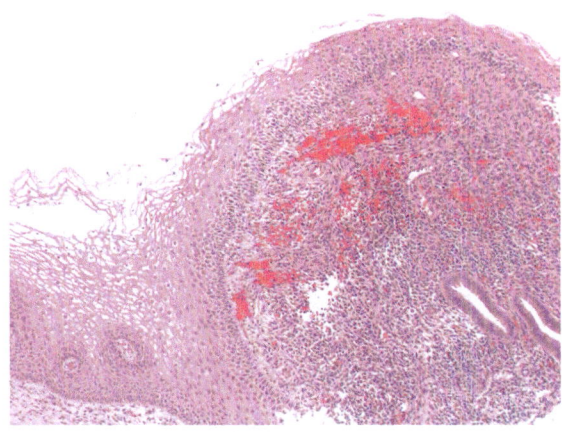

FIG. 5.2 Surface squamous epithelium covers an endometriotic nodule of cellular endometrial stroma with embedded endometrial glands; low power, hematoxylin and eosin stain

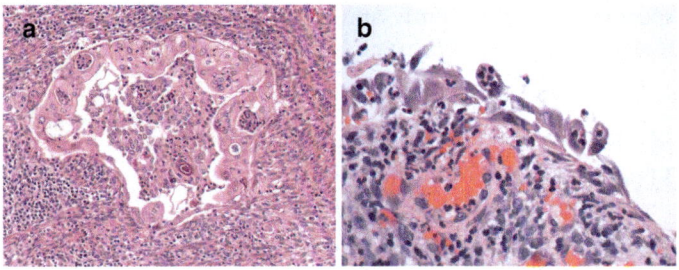

FIG. 5.3 (**a**) The gland-lining cells of oxyphil metaplasia have abundant pink cytoplasm and are associated with inflammatory cells; medium power, hematoxylin and eosin stain. (**b**) An example of oxyphil metaplasia covering an endocervical polyp is depicted; high power, hematoxylin and eosin stain

eosinophilic, and focally vacuolated cytoplasm and enlarged slightly irregular nuclei (Fig. 5.3) [4]. This metaplasia is akin to the eosinophilic change noted in endometrium where it is thought to be a reaction to degeneration or breakdown.

Ectopic prostatic tissue has rarely been identified in the cervix [5–7]. The prostatic glands have a two-cell layer lining,

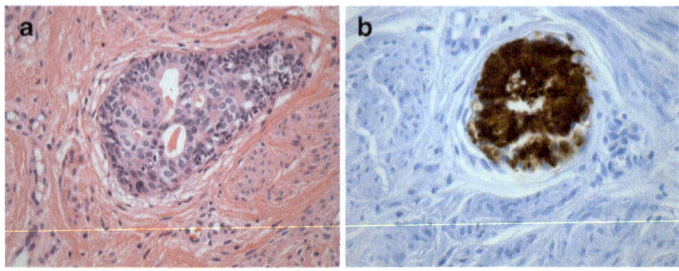

FIG. 5.4 (**a**) A nodule of ectopic prostate is made up of cells with small central round nuclei, amphophilic cytoplasm and eosinophilic luminal material; high power, hematoxylin and eosin stain. (**b**) Immunohistochemical staining for prostatic-specific antigen is positive in ectopic prostatic glands; medium power

flattened cells next to the basement membrane and columnar cells facing the lumen (Fig. 5.4). Most lesions are positive for prostatic-specific acid phosphatase and in many cases, prostatic-specific antigen. Recently an origin from Skene's glands, the female equivalent of prostate glands, has been proposed [8].

# Histology of Endocervical Glandular Hyperplasia

Tunnel clusters are aggregates of endocervical glands lined by tall columnar epithelium which form rounded subsurface masses (type A) [9]. The glands may become cystic with more flattened epithelium (type B) (Fig. 5.5). Reactive atypia of the glandular epithelium may occur [10].

Microglandular hyperplasia (MGH) consists of closely packed small glands which are lined by cells showing distinctive subnuclear vacuoles (Fig. 5.6). MGH is often noted in endocervical polyps (ECPs) and is common in women treated with hormones such as contraceptives. Rarely, atypia in MGH may simulate carcinoma [11].

Endocervical glandular hyperplasia is rare and may occur either as a diffuse band-like proliferation of endocervical

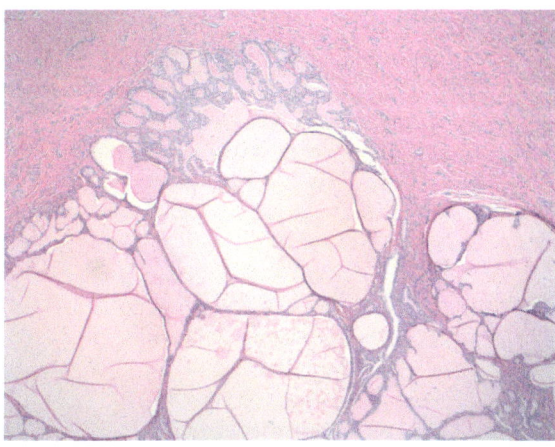

FIG. 5.5 Tunnel clusters at low power are composed of variably dilated tightly clustered glands near the mucosal surface of the cervix; low power, hematoxylin and eosin stain

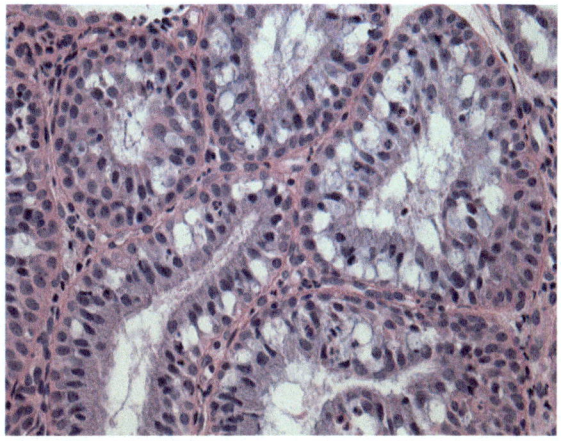

FIG. 5.6 Subnuclear vacuoles are characteristic of microglandular hyperplasia of endocervical glands; medium power, hematoxylin and eosin stain

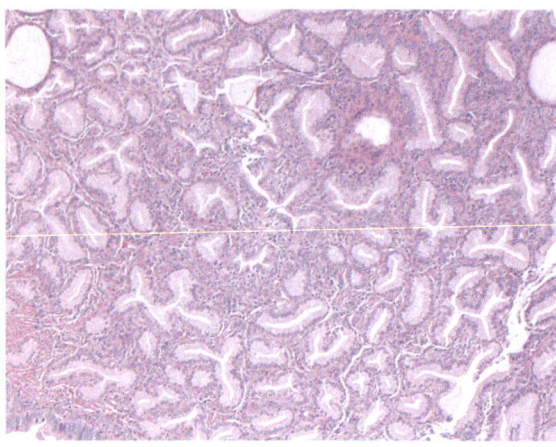

FIG. 5.7 Tightly packed otherwise normal-appearing endocervical glands characterize endocervical glandular hyperplasia; medium power, hematoxylin and eosin stain

glands known as diffuse laminar endocervical glandular hyperplasia (DEGH) or as lobular endocervical hyperplasia (LEGH) (Fig. 5.7). DEGH is composed of a superficial band of tightly packed benign-appearing endocervical glands. LEGH is made up of a lobular arrangement of tightly packed glands showing pyloric gland metaplasia. Some have suggested that LEGH is a precursor lesion to mucinous endocervical adenocarcinoma.

Mesonephric hyperplasia is characterized by small round tubules lined by low cuboidal non-mucinous epithelium with dense intraluminal eosinophilic material (Fig. 5.8) [12, 13]. While the uncommon mesonephric remnants are most commonly found in the deep lateral wall of the cervix, the even less common mesonephric hyperplasia can extend throughout the cervical wall to the luminal surface [14–16].

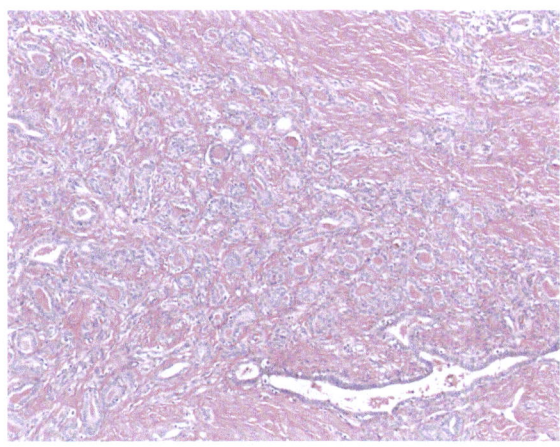

FIG. 5.8 Mesonephric hyperplasia usually occurs deep in the cervical wall but can extend to the mucosal surface. The round glands often contain dense rounded eosinophilic material. Occasionally a mesonephric duct will be associated with the gland proliferation as seen in the *lower right* of the image; low power, hematoxylin and eosin stain

# Histology of Reactive, Infectious, and Inflammatory Lesions

Reactive atypia has been described in normal endocervical glands and surface glandular epithelium secondary to trauma, such as endocervical or endometrial curettage, infectious organisms, or radiation therapy (Fig. 5.9) [17].

Viral infections of the endocervical epithelium, especially with cytomegalovirus and Herpes simplex virus, can cause reactive atypia [18, 19].

Pregnancy may cause endocervical atypia, especially the Arias-Stella reaction (Fig. 5.10) [20].

Finally, endocervical atypia maybe found in ECPs, most likely secondary to traumatization of the surface of the lesion (Fig. 5.11) [21].

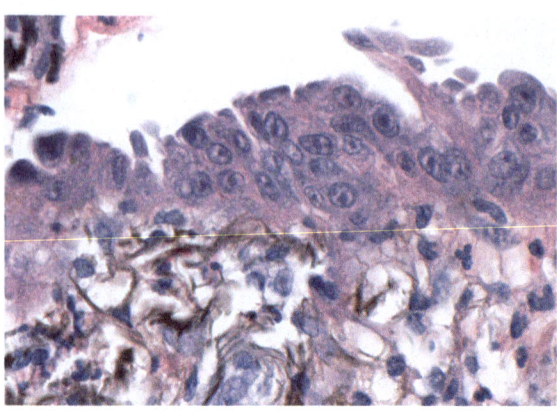

FIG. 5.9 Reactive endocervical epithelium shows nuclear enlargement with variation in nuclear size and frequently prominent nucleoli; high power, hematoxylin and eosin stain

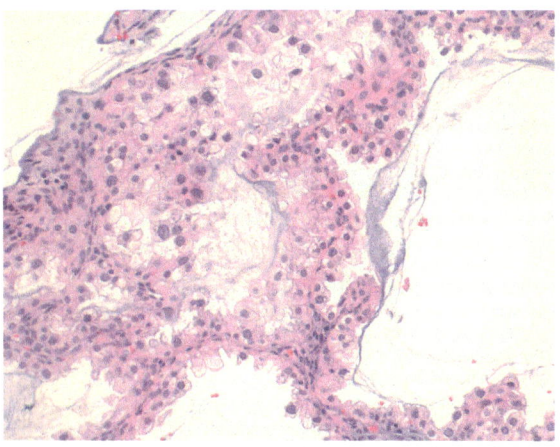

FIG. 5.10 The Arias-Stella reaction is made up of glands with an undulating luminal outline and cells with dark, smudgy, enlarged nuclei and delicate, clear cytoplasm; medium power, hematoxylin and eosin stain

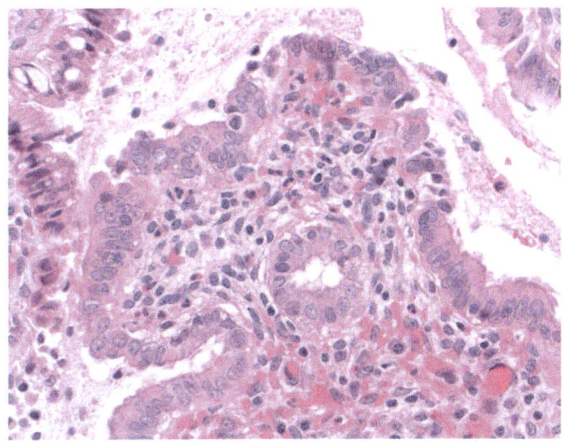

FIG. 5.11 Cervical epithelium adjacent to a biopsy site covered by markedly reactive, enlarged endocervical cells; high power, hematoxylin and eosin stain

In addition to true reactive changes of the endocervical mucosa, endocervical sampling devices (brooms and brushes) that reach high into the canal and scrape large numbers of cells from the epithelium may cause diagnostic difficulties for cytologists. The presence of large aggregates of densely packed endocervical cells (the so-called hyperchromatic crowded groups (HCGs)) can lead to over interpretation as "atypical," primarily because of the normal pleomorphism of native endocervical cells and because of the nuclear hyperchromasia associated with extreme cell overlap in such lesions.

# Cytology of Reactive Endocervical Cells and Repair

**Features:**
- Enlarged nuclei
- Enlarged nucleoli
- Uniform chromatin

- Euchromasia
- Smooth nuclear membrane
- In repair, cell groups resemble "taffy pull" or "school of fish"

Typical reactive changes in endocervical cells occur under a variety of circumstances, including trauma, infectious or inflammatory processes, and chronic irritation; however, the causes of these changes are often obscure. The nuclei can become alarmingly large. The usual nuclear size is about 8 μm in diameter but the nuclei can enlarge up to 15 or 16 μm with reactive changes [22]. Nucleoli may be present and slightly enlarged (Fig. 5.12). Multinucleation may occur (Fig. 5.13). The chromatin, however, remains bland and the nuclear contour is smooth.

In addition, features of repair may be present, especially in situations such as the presence of an ECP or MGH which may protrude from the surface of the cervix and thus be prone to trauma. Although both ECP and MGH have characteristic histologic findings, the cytologic changes are not specific. Epithelial repair presents as cell culture-like flat sheets of endocervical cells with well-defined cytoplasmic

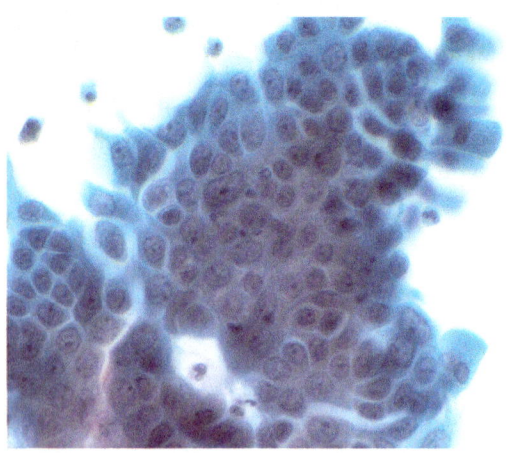

FIG. 5.12 Reactive endocervical cells with mild nuclear size variation; SurePath preparation, high power, Papanicolaou stain

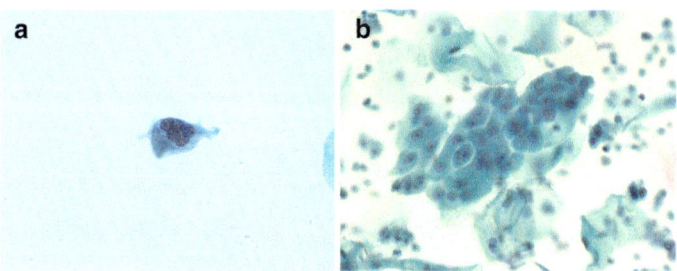

FIG. 5.13 (**a**) A single multinucleated endocervical cell; SurePath preparation, high power, Papanicolaou stain. (**b**) A sheet of mononuclear and binuclear endocervical/metaplastic repair type cells, SurePath preparation; high power, Papanicolaou stain

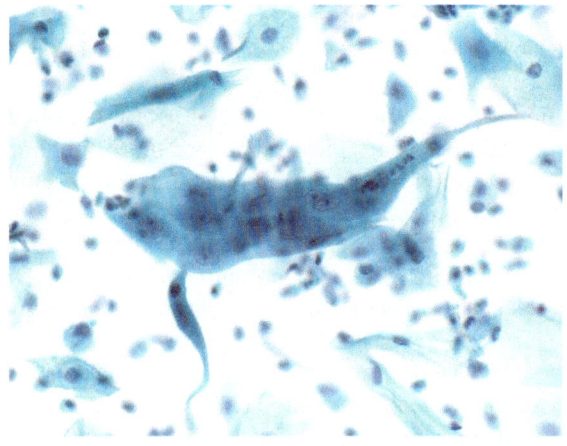

FIG. 5.14 A sheet of reparative epithelial cells with "taffy pull" appearance; SurePath preparation, high power, Papanicolaou stain

boundaries giving the sheet a cobblestone appearance (Fig. 5.14). The cytoplasm of the cells at the periphery of the groups may appear to be stretched, as if to cover an underlying breach in the tissue, and appendages of cytoplasm from the margins of the group gives a "taffy-pull" appearance. The cells generally tend to be well polarized and can have a

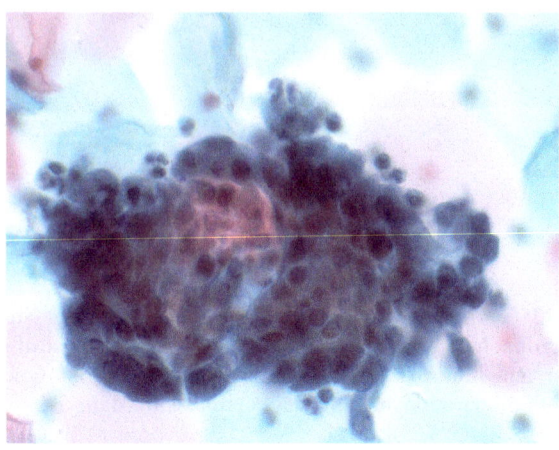

FIG. 5.15 A group of endocervical cells with a reparative swirling arrangement; SurePath preparation, high power, Papanicolaou stain

streaming effect, sometimes described as a "school of fish" pattern. The nuclei in typical repair are uniformly enlarged with open, relatively pale chromatin, with one or more distinct nucleoli and occasional mitotic figures. Reactive/reparative changes are often seen in a background of inflammation and inflammatory cells are commonly found intermixed within the sheets of reparative epithelium (Fig. 5.15).

The changes of typical repair are usually readily recognized as a benign reactive process, but if these changes become more exuberant, features of atypical repair may make differentiation from a neoplastic process more difficult. Atypical reparative epithelium shows similar architecture to typical repair, with flat sheet of cells, and polarization; however, the cells show increased nuclear pleomorphism, which can be highly bizarre with nuclear membrane irregularities, more prominent nucleoli, and chromatin abnormalities (Fig. 5.16). The differential diagnosis for atypical epithelial repair always includes invasive carcinoma, and therefore additional clues as to the true nature of the process must be sought in each case. Single abnormal glandular cells are more commonly noted in invasive carcinoma and reparative processes most commonly show a spectrum of reparative and reactive changes in sheets

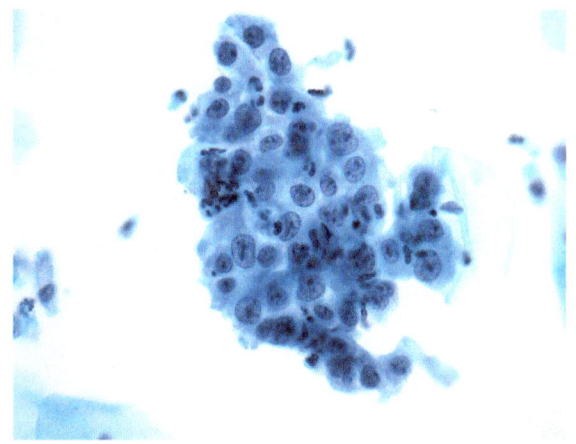

FIG. 5.16 Atypical repair in endocervical cells with large irregularly shaped nuclei and prominent nucleoli; SurePath preparation, high power, Papanicolaou stain

of cells, ranging from obviously benign to the highly atypical. The presence of background diathesis is not a good discriminator of benign and malignant as both processes may have significant underlying tissue damage. Testing for hrHPV may be of assistance in the differential diagnosis, as the vast majority (>90 %) of endocervical cancers will be positive [23]. Preparation of a cell block from the residual LBC sample may be of help as larger fragments of tissue are often found in these preparations which allow for better assessments of architecture, and can be used for special investigations [24, 25] (Fig. 5.17).

## Cytology of Tubal and Tubo-Endometrioid Metaplasia

**Features:**
- Ciliated cells
- Columnar cells with terminal bars
- Crowded cell groups

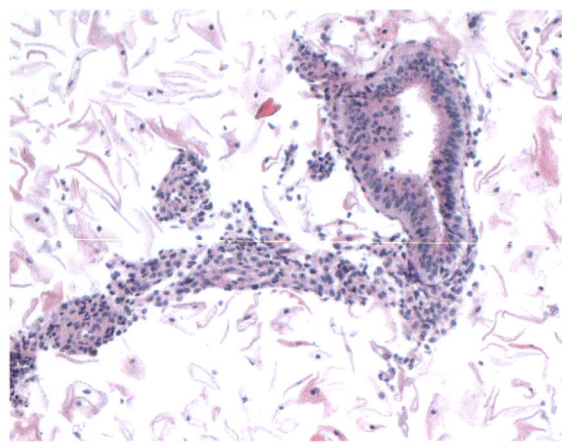

FIG. 5.17  Cell block preparation from a liquid-based cytology preparation performed to better characterize atypical glandular cells seen on cytology. The cell block section shows the presence of a lower uterine segment endometrial gland with attached stroma and surrounding squamous cells; low power, hematoxylin and eosin stain

- Nuclei small
- Chromatin uniform

In addition to squamous metaplasia, other types of metaplasia occur in the endocervical epithelium. Tubal metaplasia (TM) is characterized by the presence of two cell types, ciliated and secretory, as found lining the lumen of the fallopian tube (Fig. 5.18). TM has been reported to be common and is not related to physiologic or preneoplastic conditions [26]. On cytology, TM will appear as HCG of glandular cells, with generally uniformly small nuclei. The major key to recognition of TM is identification of cilia and/or terminal bars, although many cases do not show this feature (Fig. 5.19). In such cases, reliance on other features, including smooth, nongranular chromatin, and the lack of mitotic figures, apoptotic bodies, and prominent nucleoli should assist in a correct interpretation.

TEM is characterized by the presence of pseudostratified columnar cells with a relatively high nuclear to cytoplasmic

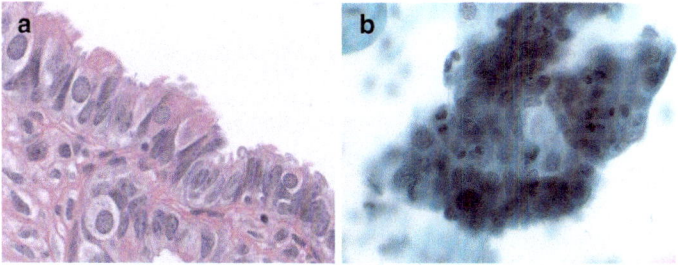

FIG. 5.18  (**a**) A histologic section of fallopian tube mucosa showing ciliated cells and non-ciliated cells; high power, hematoxylin and eosin stain. (**b**) On cytology, tubal metaplasia presents as crowded glandular cells with cilia; SurePath preparation, high power, Papanicolaou stain

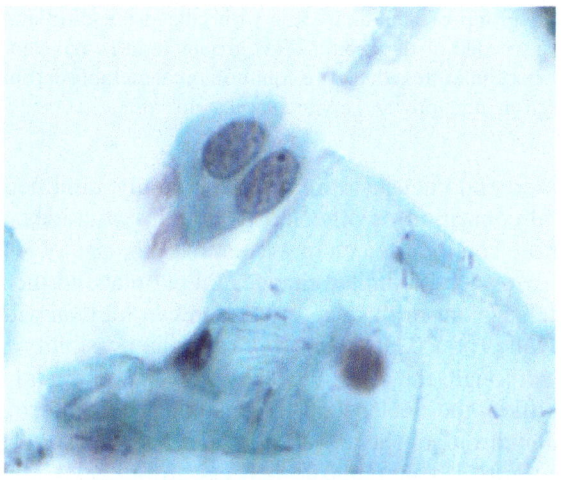

FIG. 5.19  A pair of endocervical cells with cilia attached to the terminal bar in the luminal aspect of the cell; SurePath preparation, high power, Papanicolaou stain

ratio, some with cilia similar to fallopian tube epithelium and some with apical blebs similar to endometrial glandular cells, but without associated endometrial stroma as is seen in endometriosis. The cytoplasm of the cells lacks the delicate mucin droplets seen in the usual type of endocervical cell (Fig. 5.20).

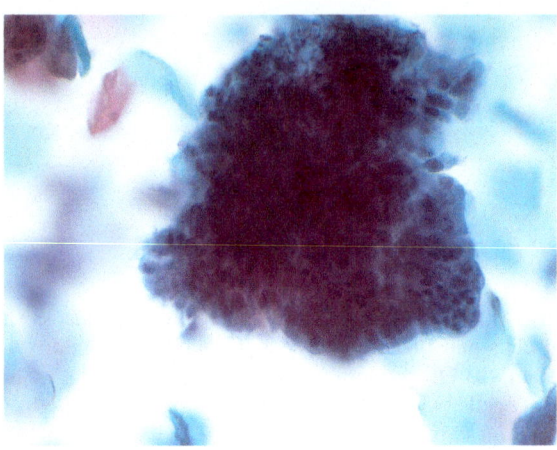

Fɪɢ. 5.20 Tubo-endometrioid metaplasia (TEM) presents as a crowded group of glandular cells with cilia protruding along the entire free edge of the group; TEM groups tend to be even larger and more cellular than the more common tubal metaplasia; SurePath preparation, high power, Papanicolaou stain

TEM and endometriosis are most commonly identified after cervical conization or other posttraumatic situations, and is also more commonly seen in women over the age of 30 years, as an extension of similar changes taking place in the lower uterine segment in this age group. On cytology, as with TM, TEM will produce HCG that will raise the possibility of AIS [27]. Although the cells in TEM are crowded and pseudostratified, the nuclei tend to be small with uniform, nongranular chromatin. Scattered ciliated cells are very helpful in recognition of a metaplastic process; however, it is always important to remember that TM is common and can therefore coexist with neoplastic conditions, so each group or cell identified must be evaluated individually.

Endometriosis in the cervix may be visible to the clinician as one or more small, blue or red nodules on the exocervix. On cytology, endometriosis cannot be distinguished from LUS sampling, and therefore clinical correlation should aid in a correct interpretation.

# Cytology of Pregnancy-Induced Changes

**Features:**
- Enlarged endocervical cells
- Hypervacuolated glandular cells
- Decidual cells—large, mononuclear, dark nuclei, dense cytoplasm

Under the influence of the hormones of pregnancy, the endocervical glandular cells become enlarged [22]. In addition, the endocervix may be everted leading to increased sampling of endocervical cells. Rarely more specific findings of pregnancy may be identified and may be mistaken for abnormal endocervical cells. Trophoblast cells, the advance guard of the developing placenta, are large mononuclear cells with very hyperchromatic, irregularly shaped nuclei (Fig. 5.21).

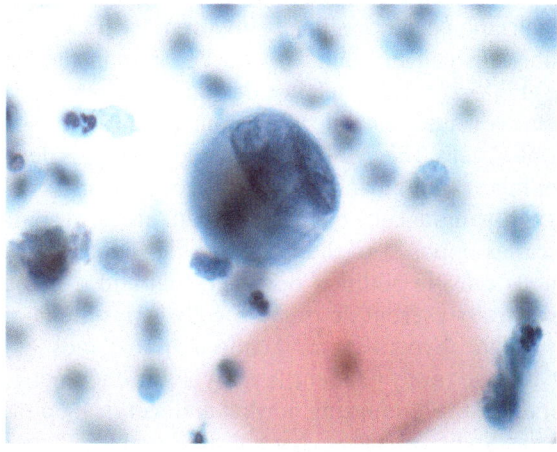

Fig. 5.21 A single very large round cell in a pregnant patient suggestive of a trophoblast cell; usually only one such cell will be found in a cervical cytology sample limiting the ability to pursue confirmatory testing (e.g., human placental lactogen and keratin immunocytochemical staining); SurePath preparation, high power, Papanicolaou stain

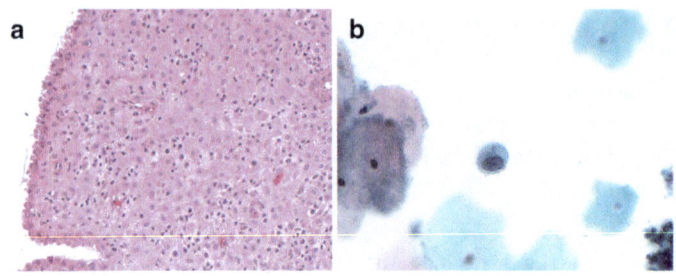

Fig. 5.22 (a) A histologic section of decidualized endocervix with *large round pink* cells filling the stroma; hematoxylin and eosin stain, medium power. (b) A single small epithelioid cell with a central nucleus presumed to be a decidual cell identified in cervical cytology from a pregnant woman; SurePath preparation, high power, Papanicolaou stain

The process of decidualization is characterized by large cells which are usually confined to the endometrial stroma. Decidualization can occasionally involve the cervix and hence decidual cells can be found in the Pap test in this circumstance (Fig. 5.22). The nuclei of decidual cells are very large but more vesicular and pale when compared to those of cytotrophoblast cells. The cytoplasm of decidual cells is dense and eosinophilic, often having an appearance similar to keratinization in squamous cells, but decidual cells are most commonly spherical as opposed to the pleomorphic shapes noted with squamous cells. In addition both decidual and trophoblastic cells generally present as isolated cells. Arias-Stella change occurs in the hypersecretory endometrial glands of pregnancy and can rarely be identified involving endometriosis of the cervix or even replacing normal endocervical epithelium. The Arias-Stella change is characterized by large hypervacuolated glandular cells with hyperchromatic, irregular nuclei protruding into the gland lumen (Fig. 5.23). Although unlikely, any of these pregnancy-associated cells may be found rarely in the cervical cytology sample obtained at the first prenatal visit. While distinguishing one entity from the other is diffi-

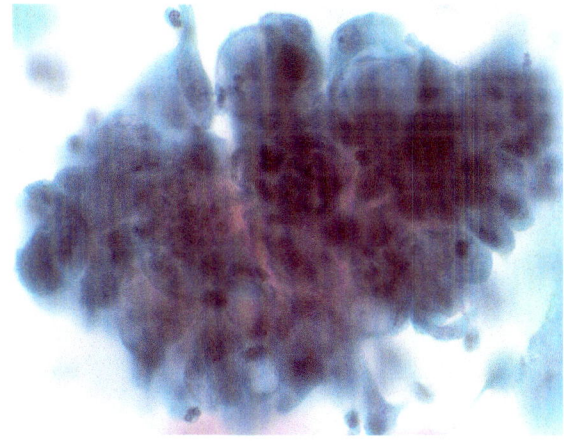

FIG. 5.23 A large hypervacuolated group of glandular cells in pregnancy is the equivalent of Arias-Stella change seen on histology, SurePath preparation, high power, Papanicolaou stain

cult on cytology, one should always be aware of these types of physiologic changes that occur during pregnancy and can be seen in cervical cytology specimens [28]. Raising this differential diagnosis and looking carefully for the specific types of differentiation noted above, and correlating the clinical information should assist in arriving at a correct interpretation.

# Cytology of Changes Due to Intrauterine Device

**Features:**
- Tangled mass of filamentous *Actinomyces* bacteria
- Glandular cell clusters with large cytoplasmic vacuoles
- Single mononuclear cells with high nuclear to cytoplasmic ratio

The presence of an intrauterine device (IUD) is well known to cause changes in squamous cells, endocervical and

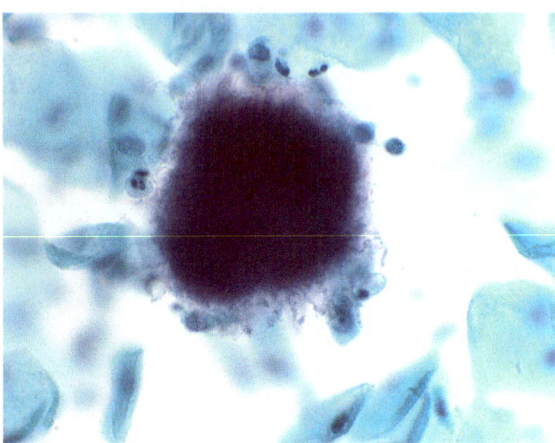

Fig. 5.24 Clusters of filamentous bacteria consistent with Actinomyces are often a clue to the presence of an IUD; SurePath preparation, high power, Papanicolaou stain

endometrial glands presumably due to irritation by the IUD in the endometrial cavity and the attached string that exits the uterus through the endocervical canal. Probably the most common finding is tangled masses of *Actinomyces* bacteria which according to one study are present in 25 % of cervical cytology samples from women using an IUD (Fig. 5.24) [29]. Rare relatively small single epithelial cells with high nuclear to cytoplasmic ratios can exfoliate and mimic the cells of HSIL (Fig. 5.25). The IUD can also cause degenerative changes and sloughing of high endocervical cells or cells from the LUS which exfoliate as three-dimensional clusters of hypervacuolated cells [30] (Fig. 5.26a). The vacuoles are large and pleomorphic and have been referred to as "bubble gum" vacuoles because of their characteristic configurations at the margins of the groups. If the presence of the IUD is not revealed in the history or if the tell tale sign of *Actinomyces* is not present, the cytologist may be compelled to interpret

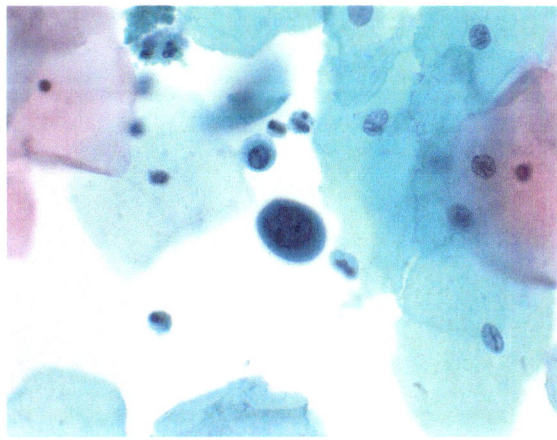

Fig. 5.25 This single epithelial cell with dense cytoplasm and a high nuclear to cytoplasmic ratio is a change noted to occur in women using an IUD and mimics cells of HSIL; SurePath preparation, high power, Papanicolaou stain

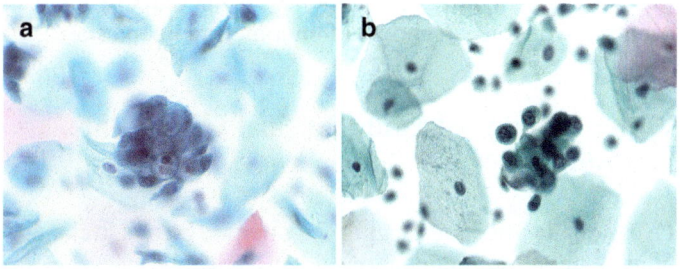

Fig. 5.26 Changes secondary to the presence of an IUD include (**a**) hypervacuolated endocervical cells and (**b**) both vacuolated cells and a single atypical cell; SurePath preparation, high power, Papanicolaou stain

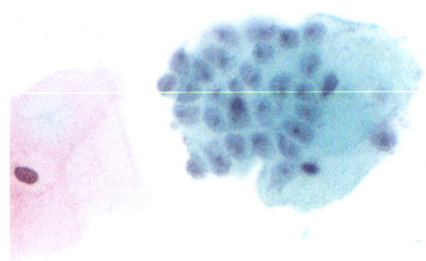

FIG. 5.27 Trichomonads are usually identified as single organisms but when clustered, the group can resemble atypical endocervical cells; SurePath preparation, high power, Papanicolaou stain

the single cells as at least ASC-H and the hypervacuolated glandular cells as atypical glandular cells, NOS (Fig. 5.26b). The presence of IUDs in women over 40 years of age can prompt erroneous diagnoses of endometrial neoplasia.

## Other Mimics of Endocervical Glandular Neoplasia

Occasionally infectious agents can provoke cytologic changes mimicking atypical endocervical cells. Trichomonads, a common infectious parasite identified in cervical cytology, are usually present singly but can form groups that may resemble endocervical glandular cells (Fig. 5.27). Herpes simplex usually is recognized when the viral cytopathic effect is florid (Fig. 5.28a) but early nuclear changes can mimic endocervical glandular atypia (Fig. 5.28b).

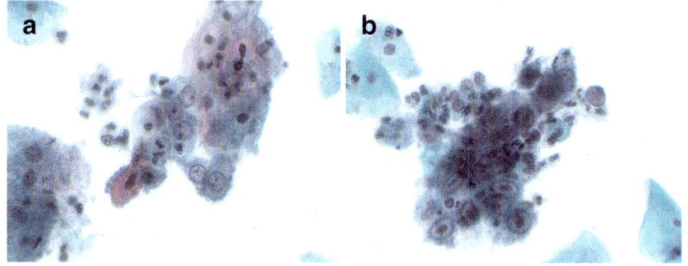

Fig. 5.28 The presence of Herpes simplex virus (HSV) can cause atypia of endocervical nuclei (**a**) which may resemble epithelial repair; fully developed HSV cytopathic effect elsewhere on the cytology sample (ground glass chromatin in the *upper right* and Cowdry A inclusions in cells in the *lower left*) confirms the true nature of the atypia (**b**), ThinPrep preparation, high power, Papanicolaou stain

# References

1. Young RH, Clement PB. Endocervical adenocarcinoma and its variants: their morphology and differential diagnosis. Histopathology. 2002;41(3):185–207.
2. Babkowski RC, Wilbur DC, Rutkowski MA, Facik MS, Bonfiglio TA. The effects of endocervical canal topography, tubal metaplasia, and high canal sampling on the cytologic presentation of nonneoplastic endocervical cells. Am J Clin Pathol. 1996;105(4):403–10.
3. Oliva E, Clement PB, Young RH. Tubal and tubo-endometrioid metaplasia of the uterine cervix. Unemphasized features that may cause problems in differential diagnosis: a report of 25 cases. Am J Clin Pathol. 1995;103(5):618–23.
4. Jones MA, Young RH. Atypical oxyphilic metaplasia of the endocervical epithelium: a report of six cases. Int J Gynecol Pathol. 1997;16(2):99–102.
5. Larraza-Hernandez O, Molberg KH, Lindberg G, Albores-Saavedra J. Ectopic prostatic tissue in the uterine cervix. Int J Gynecol Pathol. 1997;16(3):291–3.
6. Nucci MR, Ferry JA, Young RH. Ectopic prostatic tissue in the uterine cervix: a report of four cases and review of ectopic prostatic tissue. Am J Surg Pathol. 2000;24(9):1224–30.

7. McCluggage WG, Ganesan R, Hirschowitz L, Miller K, Rollason TP. Ectopic prostatic tissue in the uterine cervix and vagina: report of a series with a detailed immunohistochemical analysis. Am J Surg Pathol. 2006;30(2):209–15.

8. Kelly P, McBride HA, Kennedy K, Connolly LE, McCluggage WG. Misplaced Skene's glands: glandular elements in the lower female genital tract that are variably immunoreactive with prostate markers and that encompass vaginal tubulosquamous polyp and cervical ectopic prostatic tissue. Int J Gynecol Pathol. 2011;30(6):605–12.

9. Fluhmann CF. Focal hyperplasis (tunnel clusters) of the cervix uteri. Obstet Gynecol. 1961;17:206–14.

10. Jones MA, Young RH. Endocervical type A (noncystic) tunnel clusters with cytologic atypia. A report of 14 cases. Am J Surg Pathol. 1996;20(11):1312–8.

11. Young RH, Scully RE. Atypical forms of microglandular hyperplasia of the cervix simulating carcinoma. A report of five cases and review of the literature. Am J Surg Pathol. 1989;13(1):50–6.

12. Ferry JA, Scully RE. Mesonephric remnants, hyperplasia, and neoplasia in the uterine cervix. A study of 49 cases. Am J Surg Pathol. 1990;14(12):1100–11.

13. Seidman JD, Tavassoli FA. Mesonephric hyperplasia of the uterine cervix: a clinicopathologic study of 51 cases. Int J Gynecol Pathol. 1995;14(4):293–9.

14. Jones MA, Andrews J, Tarraza HM. Mesonephric remnant hyperplasia of the cervix: a clinicopathologic analysis of 14 cases. Gynecol Oncol. 1993;49(1):41–7.

15. Welsh T, Fu YS, Chan J, Brundage HA, Rutgers JL. Mesonephric remnants or hyperplasia can cause abnormal pap smears: a study of three cases. Int J Gynecol Pathol. 2003;22(2):121–6.

16. Hejmadi RK, Gearty JC, Waddell C, Ganesan R. Mesonephric hyperplasia can cause abnormal cervical smears: report of three cases with review of literature. Cytopathology. 2005;16(5): 240–3.

17. Scott M, Lyness RW, McCluggage WG. Atypical reactive proliferation of endocervix: a common lesion associated with endometrial carcinoma and likely related to prior endometrial sampling. Mod Pathol. 2006;19(3):470–4.

18. McGalie CE, McBride HA, McCluggage WG. Cytomegalovirus infection of the cervix: morphological observations in five cases of a possibly under-recognised condition. J Clin Pathol. 2004; 57(7):691–4.

19. Kiviat NB, Paavonen JA, Wolner-Hanssen P, Critchlow CW, Stamm WE, Douglas J, et al. Histopathology of endocervical infection caused by Chlamydia trachomatis, herpes simplex virus, Trichomonas vaginalis, and Neisseria gonorrhoeae. Hum Pathol. 1990;21(8):831–7.

20. Nucci MR, Young RH. Arias-Stella reaction of the endocervix: a report of 18 cases with emphasis on its varied histology and differential diagnosis. Am J Surg Pathol. 2004;28(5):608–12.

21. Goff BA, Atanasoff P, Brown E, Muntz HG, Bell DA, Rice LW. Endocervical glandular atypia in Papanicolaou smears. Obstet Gynecol. 1992;79(1):101–4.

22. Koss LG, Melamed MR. Koss' diagnostic cytology and its histo-pathologic bases. 5th ed. Philadelphia: Lippincott; 2006.

23. Zielinski GD, Snijders PJ, Rozendaal L, Daalmeijer NF, Risse EK, Voorhorst FJ, et al. The presence of high-risk HPV combined with specific p53 and p16INK4a expression patterns points to high-risk HPV as the main causative agent for adenocarcinoma in situ and adenocarcinoma of the cervix. J Pathol. 2003;201(4):535–43.

24. Diaz-Rosario LA, Kabawat SE. Performance of a fluid-based, thin-layer papanicolaou smear method in the clinical setting of an independent laboratory and an outpatient screening population in New England. Arch Pathol Lab Med. 1999;123(9):817–21.

25. Xing W, Hou AY, Fischer A, Owens CL, Jiang Z. The cellient automated cell block system is useful in the differential diagno-sis of atypical glandular cells in Papanicolaou tests. Cancer Cytopathol. 2014;122:8–14.

26. Jonasson JG, Wang HH, Antonioli DA, Ducatman BS. Tubal metaplasia of the uterine cervix: a prevalence study in patients with gynecologic pathologic findings. Int J Gynecol Pathol. 1992; 11(2):89–95.

27. Lundeen SJ, Horwitz CA, Larson CJ, Stanley MW. Abnormal cervicovaginal smears due to endometriosis: a continuing prob-lem. Diagn Cytopathol. 2002;26(1):35–40.

28. Kobayashi TK, Okamoto H. Cytopathology of pregnancy-induced cell patterns in cervicovaginal smears. Am J Clin Pathol. 2000;114(Suppl):S6–20.

29. Mali B, Joshi JV, Wagle U, Hazari K, Shah R, Chadha U, et al. Actinomyces in cervical smears of women using intrauterine contraceptive devices. Acta Cytol. 1986;30(4):367–71.

30. Kobayashi TK, Casslen B, Stormby N. Cytologic atypias in the uterine fluid of intrauterine contraceptive device users. Acta Cytol. 1983;27(2):138–41.

# Chapter 6
## Cytology of Endometrial Cells and Lesions

The Pap test was not designed to sample the endometrium and to screen for endometrial lesions, but endometrial cells can be identified in cervical cytology samples at a low rate that varies according to the study from a high 5 % to less than 1 % [1–3]. The presence of endometrial cells may result either from exfoliation (shedding) of the endometrium or from direct sampling. The cytologic appearance of the endometrial cells will differ between these two circumstances.

## Exfoliated Endometrium

**Features:**
Endometrial glands:
- Small cells in tightly packed three-dimensional groups
- Scant cytoplasm, although vacuoles seen if well preserved
- Chromatin dense
- Apoptotic debris

Endometrial stroma:
- Tightly compressed small cells with or without surrounding endometrial glandular cells

R.H. Tambouret and D.C. Wilbur, *Glandular Lesions of the Uterine Cervix*, Essentials in Cytopathology 19, DOI 10.1007/978-1-4939-1989-5_6, © Springer Science+Business Media New York 2015

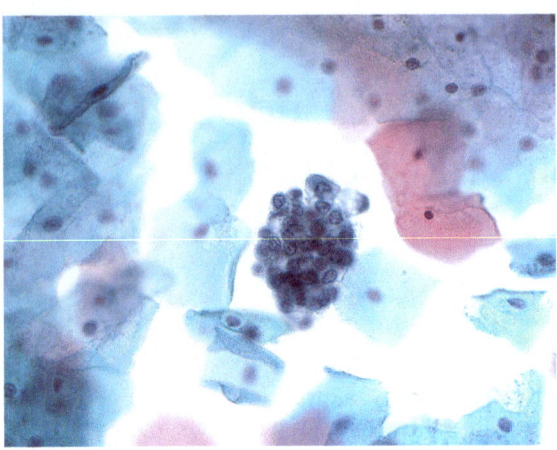

FIG. 6.1 Cluster of tightly packed small glandular cells with scant cytoplasm consistent with shed benign endometrial cells, high power, SurePath preparation, Papanicolaou stain

During the reproductive years as the menstrual cycle is completed, the endometrium is shed during menstruation and this shedding continues into the proliferative phase of the next menstrual cycle. Benign endometrial glandular and stromal cells are normally shed during the first half of the cycle and are commonly found in cervical cytology samples (Fig. 6.1). Shed cells are most commonly arranged as three-dimensional groupings because after shedding the cell groupings have time to round up while they travel down the endocervical canal before being picked up by the sampling device. Dense three-dimensional groups of clumped endometrial stroma surrounded by degenerating endometrial glandular cells are most commonly seen from day 6 to day 10 (Fig. 6.2). The dense clusters along with single small histiocytes were termed "exodus" by George Papanicolaou and their counterpart on histologic sections of endometrial biopsies are very familiar to surgical pathologists [4] (Fig. 6.3). The shed endometrial glandular cells have uniform small nuclei with inapparent to slightly more abundant vacuolated

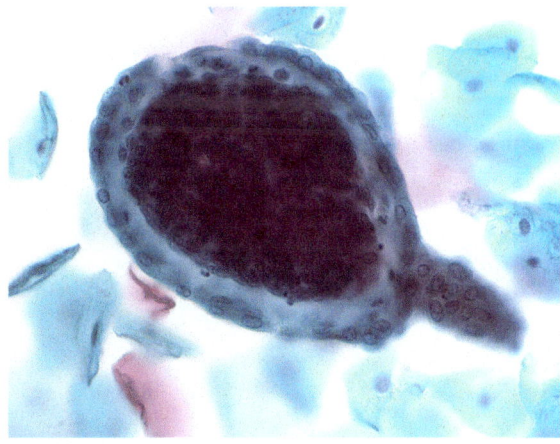

FIG. 6.2  Clusters of tightly packed stromal cells surrounded by paler endometrial glandular cells are often shed during the peak of menses, high power, SurePath preparation, Papanicolaou stain

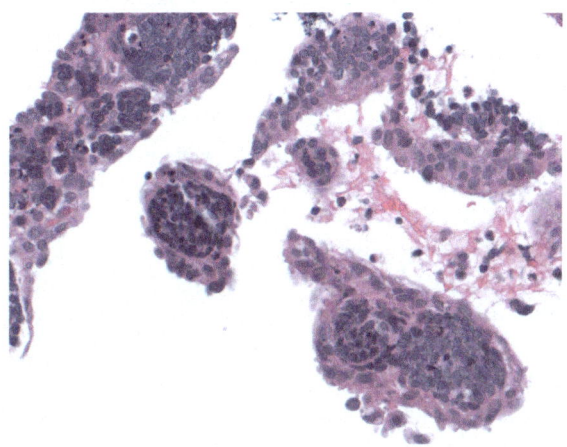

FIG. 6.3  Histologic sections of menstrual endometrium show features similar to Fig. 6.2: a tightly packed core of collapsed endometrial stroma surrounded by eosinophilic degenerating endometrial glandular epithelium, medium power, hematoxylin and eosin

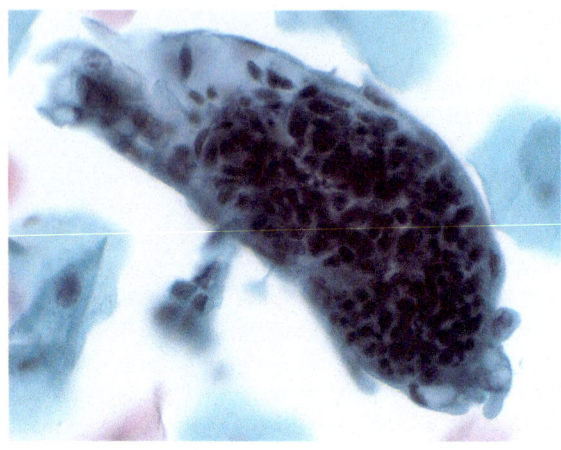

FIG. 6.4 More abundant, somewhat vacuolated cytoplasm in a stromal-glandular cluster of shed endometrium, high power, SurePath preparation, Papanicolaou stain

cytoplasm (Fig. 6.4). The increase in vacuolated cytoplasm may be due to cellular degeneration. The nuclei most commonly have a coarse granular chromatin pattern, probably a degenerative phenomenon. In addition to these familiar biphasic cell groupings, clusters made up purely of either glandular or stromal cells are also commonly noted in menstrual specimens. Apoptotic debris is often identified in clusters of glandular cells indicative of cellular breakdown (Fig. 6.5). The stromal cells, whether associated with glandular cells or present as pure groups or as single cells, are very small, with groupings in which the nuclei are tightly packed together, and have scant cytoplasm (Fig. 6.6). In the liquid-based cytology preparations, one may encounter more abundant clear cytoplasm with vacuoles, as compared to conventional smears; the difference is thought to be secondary to more rapid fixation leading to better preservation of the degenerative changes in the cells (Fig. 6.7a, b). The nuclear sizes of the cells in the SurePath samples remain small and uniform, although occasional degenerated nuclei can become quite large and hyperchromatic, a feature that can sometimes lead to erroneous

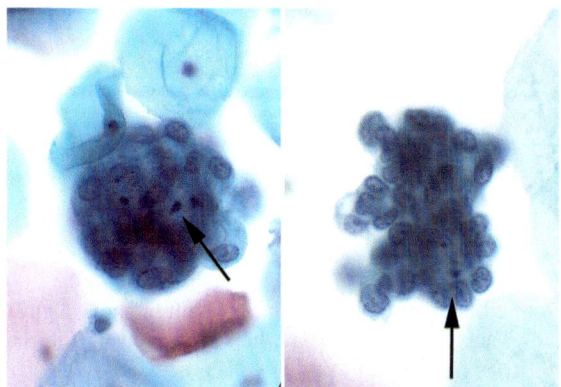

FIG. 6.5 Shed groups of endometrial glandular cells with apoptotic debris (*arrows*), high power, SurePath preparation, Papanicolaou stain

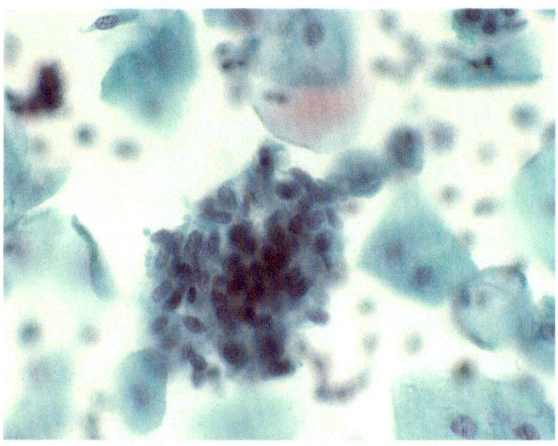

FIG. 6.6 The longer than wide nuclei in this group of shed endometrial stromal cells are well preserved; note the wispy cytoplasm and absent vacuoles high power, SurePath preparation, Papanicolaou stain

interpretations of atypia. Macrophages/histiocytes may also accompany the shed endometrium (Fig. 6.8).

According to the 2001 Bethesda System (TBS) for reporting cervical cytology, the presence of shed endometrial

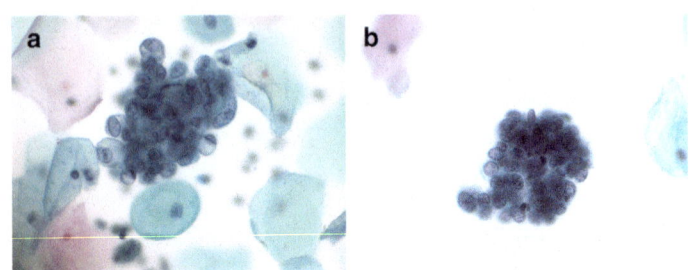

FIG. 6.7 Shed endometrial glandular cells often show slightly more abundant, vacuolated cytoplasm when processed by the SurePath method (**a**) as compared to similar cells processed by the ThinPrep method (**b**), both images, high power, SurePath preparation, Papanicolaou stain

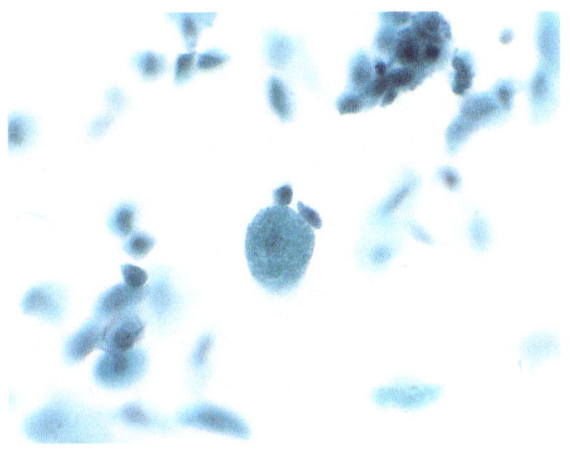

FIG. 6.8 Macrophages with abundant foamy or granular cytoplasm and round to reniform nuclei often accompany shed endometrium, high power, SurePath preparation, Papanicolaou stain

cells should not be reported in women under age 40, as this is a normal finding associated with menses. However, in women 40 and older, reporting becomes more important as benign endometrium in the cervical cytology specimen can be a marker of neoplasia, and this risk becomes greater starting at age 40 and increasing in each subsequent decade. The presence of benign-appearing endometrium in this age group is reported under the general categorization of "other" so that the clinician may correlate the finding with the patient's menstrual history. Since this reporting terminology was initiated in 2001, numerous studies have documented that the risk of endometrial neoplasm in women over 40 who are still normally menstruating is very low [2, 3, 5–8]. After menopause, however, the cytologic identification of benign endometrial cells warrants follow-up [9]. Therefore, many laboratories now only report benign-appearing endometrial cells when the patient is known to be postmenopausal or no menstrual history is given. Using this local modification of the Bethesda System terminology at Massachusetts General Hospital has decreased the number of endometrial biopsies performed without a significant loss of sensitivity for endometrial neoplasia (unpublished personal observation).

# Directly Sampled Endometrium

**Features:**
- Intact tubular glands with or without attached stroma
- Irregularly shaped fragments of stroma with small ovoid nonaligned nuclei

Directly sampled, or abraded, endometrium is present in the cervical cytology specimen when the sampling device (endocervical brush or Cervex broom™) scrapes endometrial glands and stroma from the lower uterine segment (LUS) while obtaining the endocervical sample. This can occur from vigorous sampling, but is most commonly seen in women who have undergone a prior cone biopsy or loop electrosurgical excision procedure (LEEP). The LUS is more likely to be sampled due to the foreshortened endocervical canal [10, 11]. Similarly, in patients who have undergone a trachelectomy for carcinoma of the cervix (amputation of the cervix with anastomosis of the LUS to the vagina), follow-up

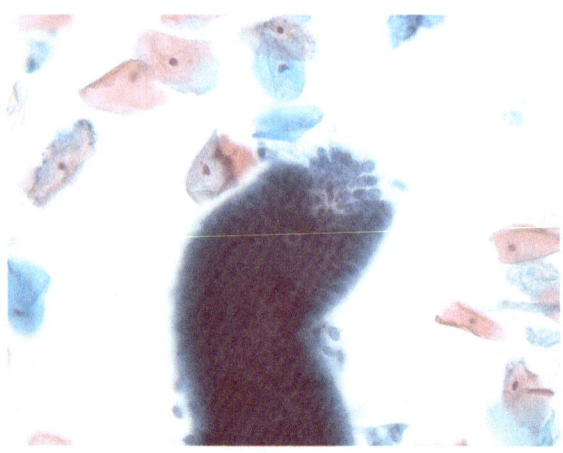

Fig. 6.9 An intact endometrial gland with a tubular shape has been pulled out of the tissue by the sampling device, medium power, SurePath preparation, Papanicolaou stain

surveillance by cytology will frequently produce abundant cells from the LUS [12].

With direct sampling, endometrial cells appear as they would in their native state, similar to what might be found on a fine needle aspiration specimen. When cells are retained in groups, the architecture is most commonly that of two-dimensionality as the groups have not had time to round up as in the shedding process described above. Intact endometrial glands are present as tubular structures with parallel sides (Fig. 6.9), or if the gland is disrupted and opened during sampling it will appear as flat honeycomb sheets of uniform cells (Fig. 6.10). Endometrial glandular cells are also present as strips of pseudostratified columnar cells when the sampling occurs in the proliferative phase, but can also show prominent single-layered vacuolated cells during the secretory phase. Cytoplasm tends to be more delicate and wispy than in shed endometrial epithelial cells. The glandular cell nuclei are uniform in size and are spaced uniformly. Mitoses and apoptotic debris may be identified during the proliferative phase (Fig. 6.11) although the LUS along with the basalis

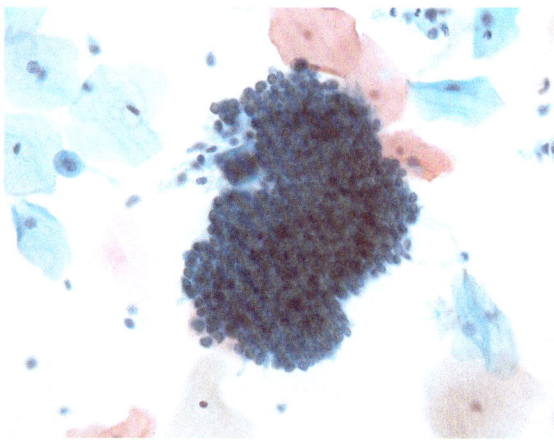

Fig. 6.10 A honeycomb sheet of small uniform endometrial glandular cells directly sampled from the tissue, high power, SurePath preparation, Papanicolaou stain

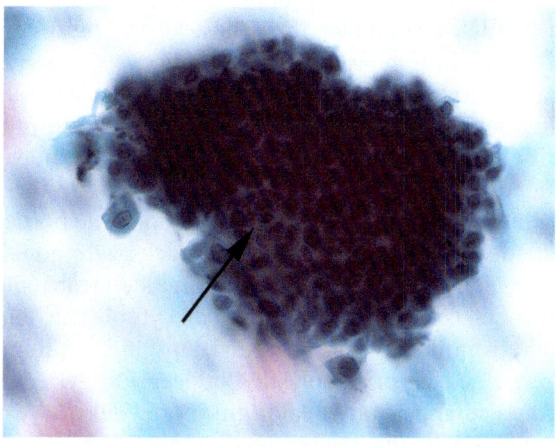

Fig. 6.11 Within a sheet of small uniform endometrial glandular cells a mitotic figure (*arrow*) is present, high power, SurePath preparation, Papanicolaou stain

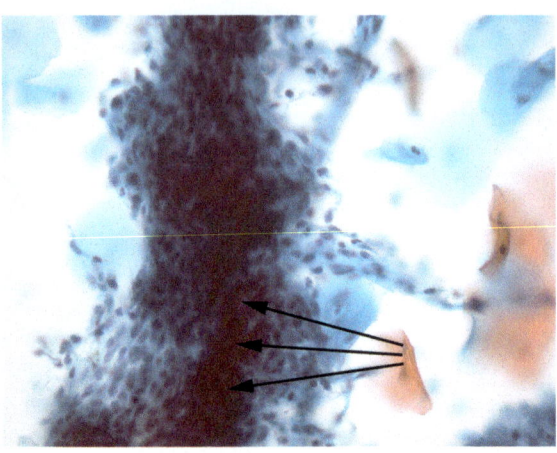

FIG. 6.12 A fragment of endometrial stroma contains an embedded blood vessel (*arrows*), high power, SurePath preparation, Papanicolaou stain

layer of the endometrium in the corpus is less responsive to the hormonal stimulation of the reproductive cycle. The presence of mitotic activity may mimic endocervical AIS, but the nuclei in LUS are smaller than those of the most common forms of AIS. In some cases, differentiation of LUS sampling from endocervical neoplasia may be difficult. Several clues favoring benign abraded endometrium include the presence of densely cellular stromal fragments which may have embedded blood vessels (Fig. 6.12) or even more revealing, intact glands (Fig. 6.13). The stromal cytoplasmic borders are ill defined and these cells have ovoid nuclei with nonaligned long axes giving the impression of a jumbled arrangement of cells. Stromal cells can often have small cytoplasmic tails that protrude from the margins of the groups and can mimic the "feathered" edges of neoplastic endocervical AIS. Stromal cells can also appear as isolated nuclei devoid of cytoplasm and sprinkled in the background of the slide (Fig. 6.14). Small epithelioid cells which are probably histiocytes may accompany the stromal cells and cell fragments. Abraded endometrial glands also will show attached stromal cells on

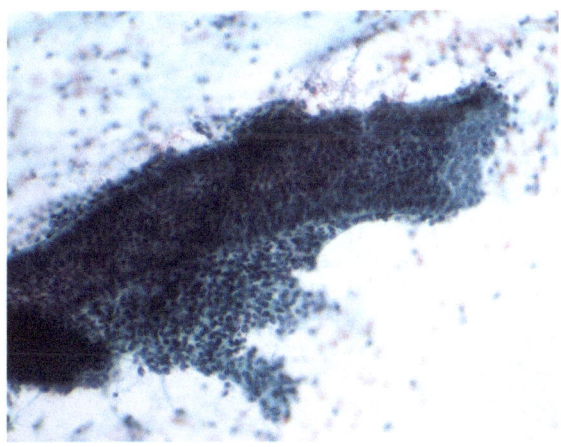

FIG. 6.13 Endometrial stroma with an intact gland has been directly sampled, low power, SurePath preparation, Papanicolaou stain

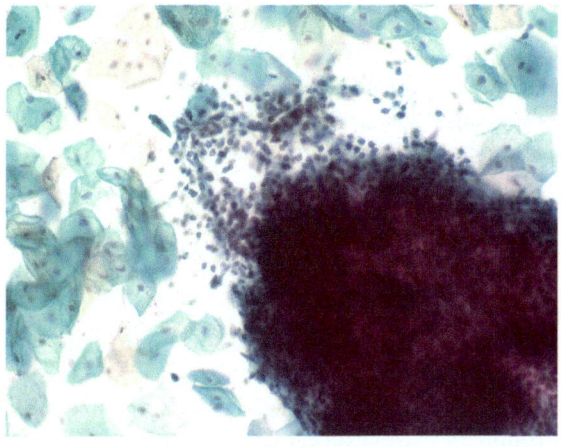

FIG. 6.14 Single stromal cells are breaking away from a large compact stromal fragment, medium power, SurePath preparation, Papanicolaou stain

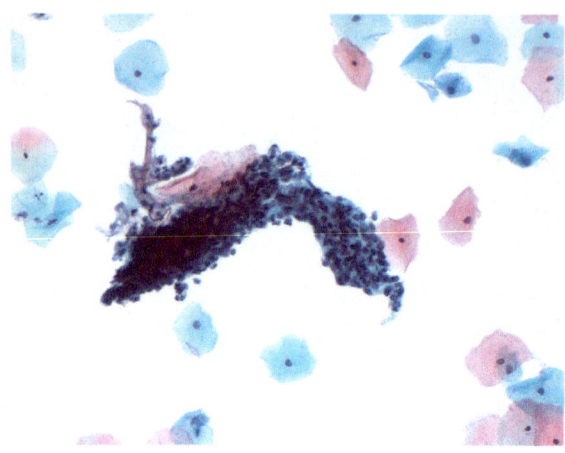

Fɪɢ. 6.15 An intact endometrial gland embedded in stromal cells; the presence of stroma helps to separate the cell group from an endocervical lesion, medium power, SurePath preparation, Papanicolaou stain

the outside surfaces of the groups, a feature not appreciated in endocervical neoplastic lesions (Fig. 6.15).

According to the 2001 TBS terminology, the presence of endometrium with the appearance of LUS as described above represents abraded endometrium and does not need to be reported, regardless of the age of the patient.

## Atypical Exfoliated Endometrial Cells

**Features:**
- Slightly enlarged glandular cells (larger than intermediate cell nuclei)
- Slight chromatin and nuclear membrane irregularities
- Prominent cytoplasmic vacuoles with or without associated neutrophils

The features of shed endometrium that merit the designation of atypical endometrial cells include nuclear enlargement,

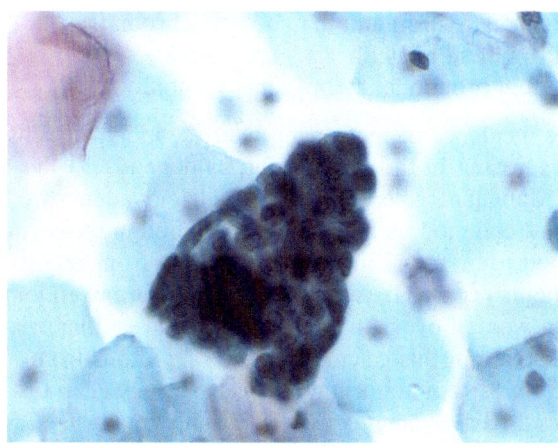

FIG. 6.16  Atypical features of this group of endometrial cells include nuclear enlargement, hyperchromasia and chromatin irregularity, high power, SurePath preparation, Papanicolaou stain

nuclear size variation, hyperchromasia, and chromatin irregularity (Fig. 6.16). The cytoplasm may be scant or more abundant and vacuolated than in completely normal-appearing endometrial cells. Three-dimensionality of the cell groups and relatively smaller nuclear size are features of atypical glandular cells that favor endometrial origin over an endocervical origin.

The frequency with which an underlying lesion is identified following the interpretation of atypical endometrial cells increases with patient age [13]. Significant pathology is identified in 17–18 % of histologic follow-up of cases reported as such [13, 14].

# Exfoliated Endometrial Adenocarcinoma

**Features:**
- Large cells in three-dimensional cell groups
- Large, irregularly shaped nuclei

- Irregular chromatin may be hypochromatic
- Prominent nucleoli
- Often prominent cytoplasmic vacuoles

The incidence of recovering overtly malignant cells from tumors arising in the uterine corpus depends on the tumor type. Malignant cells from endometrioid adenocarcinoma, the most common malignancy encountered in the corpus, are reported to be found in cervical cytology from 18.3 to 50 % of patients prior to treatment [15–17]. If normal endometrial cells in women over 40 years and atypical endometrial cells are included in this calculation, the rate varies from 37.8 to 77 % [16, 17]. An abnormal cervical cytology (Pap test) containing shed malignant cells is found in as many as 87.5 % of patients with uterine papillary serous carcinoma (UPSC) or clear cell carcinoma [17, 18].

The morphology of tumor cells depends on the tumor grade. In low grade endometrioid tumors, benign-appearing endometrial cells may be present in variable quantities (Fig. 6.17). Tumor cells may exfoliate in three-dimensional clusters with many leukocytes distending the cytoplasm

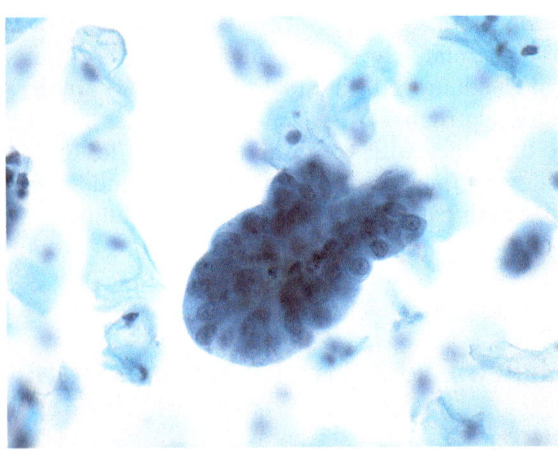

Fig. 6.17 Cluster of low grade adenocarcinoma with an orderly cellular arrangement, high power, SurePath preparation, Papanicolaou stain

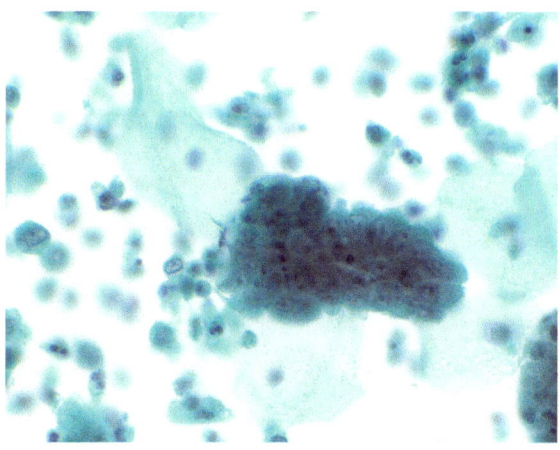

FIG. 6.18 High grade endometrial adenocarcinoma with larger more pleomorphic nuclei and a single malignant gland cell in the left of the field, high power, SurePath preparation, Papanicolaou stain

("bag of polys" appearance). Malignant epithelial cells will generally have enlarged nuclei; usually the higher the grade, the larger the nuclei. Prominent nucleoli are noted in most endometrioid adenocarcinomas, and nuclear contour irregularities may be present and even prominent in higher grade lesions. Although most shed endometrioid adenocarcinoma cells will be present in three-dimensional groupings (again a process of rounding up of cell aggregates after shedding), individual tumor cells are not uncommonly seen, particularly in higher grade lesions (Fig. 6.18). Background necrosis or diathesis, consisting of degenerated blood, fibrin and cell debris, may be identified (Fig. 6.19). Diathesis material is commonly spread thinly over the entire surface of a conventionally prepared specimen and is referred to as a "watery" diathesis. In LBC specimens, the finely granular debris tends to clump together and cling to the surface of the cells present, the so-called clinging diathesis. In addition to diathesis, large lipid-laden macrophages are often associated with endometrial malignancy (Fig. 6.20).

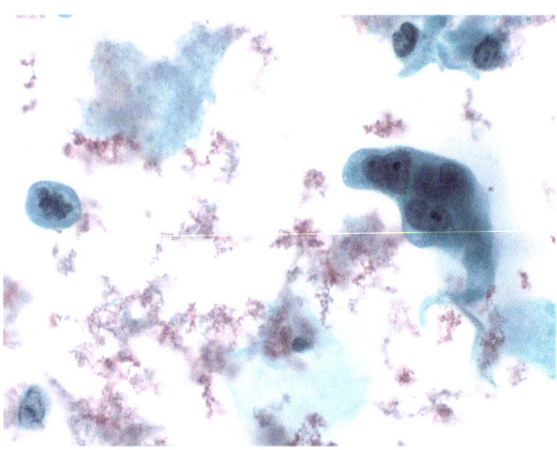

FIG. 6.19 Few cells of endometrial adenocarcinoma, one undergoing mitosis, in a background of granular acellular debris corresponding to tumor diathesis, high power, SurePath preparation, Papanicolaou stain

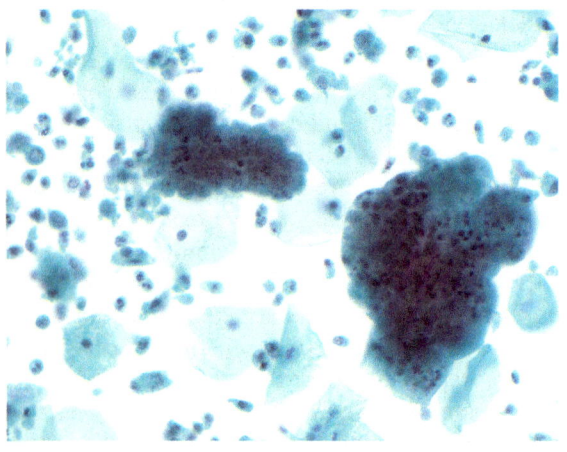

FIG. 6.20 Cluster of endometrial adenocarcinoma with associated acute inflammation within the cytoplasm; macrophages are scattered in the background, high power, SurePath preparation, Papanicolaou stain

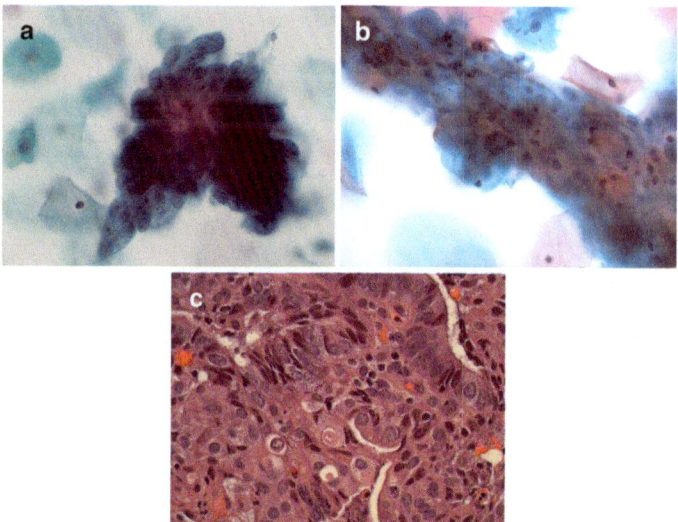

FIG. 6.21  Endometrioid adenocarcinoma (**a**) frequently is associated with squamous differentiation, high power, SurePath preparation, Papanicolaou stain; atypical squamous cells (**b**) may be identified in the cytology sample but not necessarily attached to the malignant glandular component, high power, SurePath preparation, Papanicolaou stain; the histology however (**c**) will show squamous cells arising from the malignant glands, high power, hematoxylin and eosin

Overtly malignant glandular cells in a cervical cytology sample can pose the problem of origin of the cells. Features that favor an origin from the endometrium as opposed to endocervix include three-dimensional groups of cells especially in liquid-based cytology preparations. Endocervical adenocarcinomas most commonly present as two-dimensional groups because they are directly sampled during the cytology collection procedure. On histology, endometrioid adenocarcinoma is favored when malignant glands contain foci of cells with benign squamoid differentiation; however, this feature may not be well identified on cytology specimens (Fig. 6.21). Details of the morphology of glandular lesions may be better appreciated on cell block preparations from the cytology sample [19].

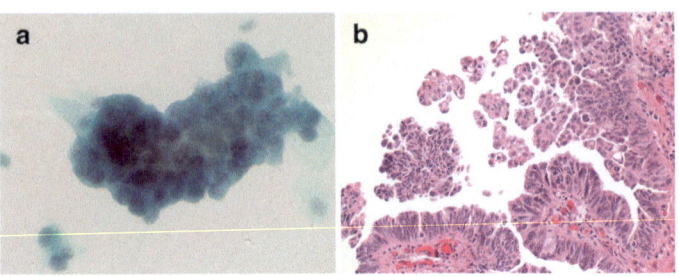

FIG. 6.22 Serous carcinoma will often present as malignant glandular cells in three-dimensional clusters (**a**); the cytology appearance correlates with the histology of detached tufts of malignant cells (**b**); image (**a**) high power, SurePath preparation, Papanicolaou stain; image (**b**) medium power, hematoxylin-eosin

Frankly malignant glandular cells have been reported to be more common in cases of UPSC than in endometrioid adenocarcinoma [17] (Fig. 6.22). Psammoma bodies are classically described with UPSC and may be associated with malignant glandular cells recovered in a cervical cytology sample (Pap test). However, the presence of psammoma bodies is not restricted to UPSC and may be found associated with benign conditions, such as mesothelial papillary hyperplasia, as well as with other papillary malignant tumors from a variety of non-gynecologic sites [20].

Carcinosarcoma (malignant mixed müllerian tumor) of the uterine corpus will often result in abnormal cytology on both conventional smears and on LBC [21,22]. Carcinosarcoma may be suspected if both carcinomatous and sarcomatous elements are present in the cytology sample; however, usually only high grade carcinoma is present (Fig. 6.23).

Other sarcomas (leiomyosarcoma and endometrial stromal sarcoma) do not usually shed cells into the cytology sample, because they do not routinely involve the endometrial surface. Low grade endometrial stromal sarcoma has been reportedly identified on cytology where the challenge can be to distinguish the tumor cells from normal endometrial stroma.

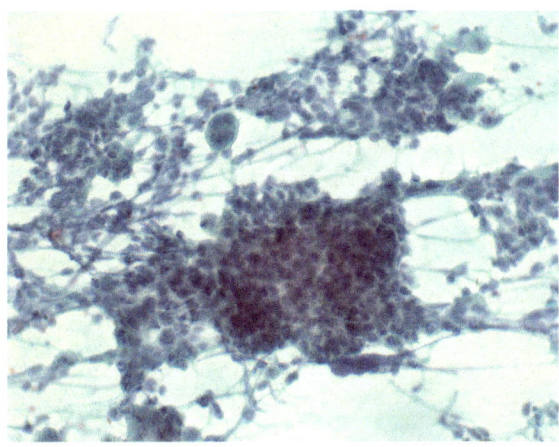

FIG. 6.23 Carcinosarcoma of the uterine corpus may shed high grade poorly cohesive malignant cells and large pleomorphic epithelioid cells, medium power, SurePath preparation, Papanicolaou stain

## Post-hysterectomy Vaginal Smears Following Surgery for Malignancy

Post-hysterectomy vaginal smears are commonly performed every 6 months for 2 years following surgical removal of the uterus for endometrial adenocarcinoma. Usually only squamous epithelial cells are obtained but occasionally benign endocervical-type glandular cells may be identified (Fig. 6.24) [23]. The benign glandular cells result from a metaplastic change in vaginal epithelium, but their presence may cause concern for recurrent endometrial adenocarcinoma in the vaginal vault. Generally, recurrent tumor shows malignant cytologic features (Fig. 6.25a) and may be associated with tumor diathesis (Fig. 6.25b). Comparison with original cytologic or histologic malignant samples may be helpful in clarifying the process.

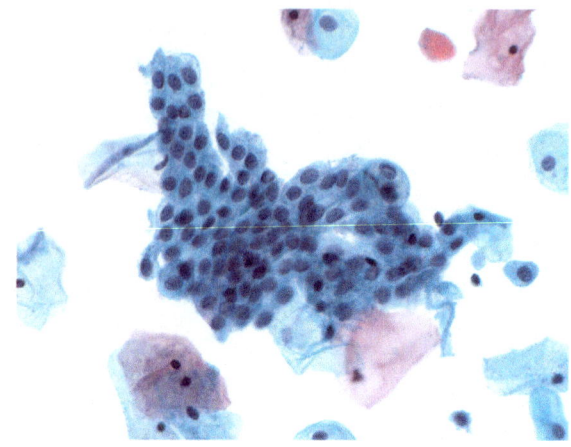

FIG. 6.24  A flat sheet of benign-appearing endocervical-like cells in a post-hysterectomy vaginal sample, high power, SurePath preparation, Papanicolaou stain

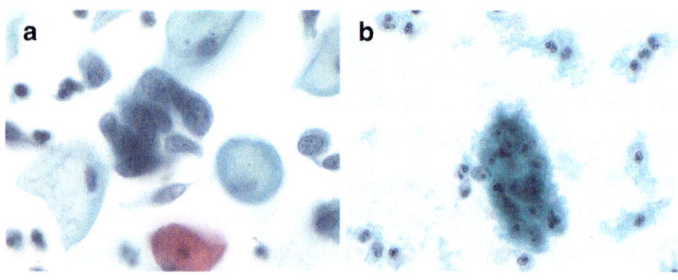

FIG. 6.25  Recurrent adenocarcinoma in a vaginal sample obtained as follow-up post-hysterectomy. (**a**) Glandular cells with abnormally clumped chromatin and irregular nuclear contours are consistent with malignancy; (**b**) tumor diathesis surrounds malignant glandular cells; both images, high power, SurePath preparation, Papanicolaou stain

# References

1. Greenspan DL, Cardillo M, Davey DD, Heller DS, Moriarty AT. Endometrial cells in cervical cytology: review of cytological features and clinical assessment. J Low Genit Tract Dis. 2006;10(2):111–22.

2. Moroney JW, Zahn CM, Heaton RB, Crothers B, Kendall BS, Elkas JC. Normal endometrial cells in liquid-based cervical cytology specimens in women aged 40 or older. Gynecol Oncol. 2007;105(3):672–6.

3. Thrall M, Kjeldahl K, Gulbahce HE, Pambuccian SE. Liquid-based Papanicolaou test (SurePath) interpretations before histologic diagnosis of endometrial hyperplasias and carcinomas: study of 272 cases classified by the 2001 Bethesda system. Cancer. 2007;111(4):217–23.

4. Koprowska I, George N. Papanicolaou living memories, monuments, and archives. Diagn Cytopathol. 1985;1(1):68–72.

5. Simsir A, Carter W, Elgert P, Cangiarella J. Reporting endometrial cells in women 40 years and older: assessing the clinical usefulness of Bethesda 2001. Am J Clin Pathol. 2005;123(4):571–5.

6. Aslan DL, Crapanzano JP, Harshan M, Erroll M, Vakil B, Pirog EC. The Bethesda System 2001 recommendation for reporting of benign appearing endometrial cells in Pap tests of women age 40 years and older leads to unwarranted surveillance when followed without clinical qualifiers. Gynecol Oncol. 2007;107(1): 86–93.

7. Beal HN, Stone J, Beckmann MJ, McAsey ME. Endometrial cells identified in cervical cytology in women > or = 40 years of age: criteria for appropriate endometrial evaluation. Am J Obstet Gynecol. 2007;196(6):568.e1–5; discussion 568.e5–6.

8. Kapali M, Agaram NP, Dabbs D, Kanbour A, White S, Austin RM. Routine endometrial sampling of asymptomatic premenopausal women shedding normal endometrial cells in Papanicolaou tests is not cost effective. Cancer. 2007;111(1):26–33.

9. Brogi E, Tambouret R, Bell DA. Classification of benign endometrial glandular cells in cervical smears from postmenopausal women. Cancer. 2002;96(2):60–6.

10. de Peralta-Venturino MN, Purslow MJ, Kini SR. Endometrial cells of the "lower uterine segment" (LUS) in cervical smears obtained by endocervical brushings: a source of potential diagnostic pitfall. Diagn Cytopathol. 1995;12(3):263–8; discussion 268–71.

11. Heaton Jr RB, Harris TF, Larson DM, Henry MR. Glandular cells derived from direct sampling of the lower uterine segment in patients status post-cervical cone biopsy. A diagnostic dilemma. Am J Clin Pathol. 1996;106(4):511–6.

12. Sauder K, Wilbur DC, Duska L, Tambouret RH. An approach to post-radical trachelectomy vaginal-isthmus cytology. Diagn Cytopathol. 2009;37(6):437–42.

13. Zhao C, Austin RM, Pan J, Barr N, Martin SE, Raza A, et al. Clinical significance of atypical glandular cells in conventional pap smears in a large, high-risk U.S. west coast minority population. Acta Cytol. 2009;53(2):153–9.

14. Zhou J, Tomashefski Jr JF, Sawady J, Ferrer H, Khiyami A. The diagnostic value of the ThinPrep pap test in endometrial carcinoma: a prospective study with histological follow-up. Diagn Cytopathol. 2013;41(5):408–12.

15. Larson DM, Copeland LJ, Gallager HS, Gershenson DM, Freedman RS, Wharton JT, et al. Nature of cervical involvement in endometrial carcinoma. Cancer. 1987;59(5):959–62.

16. DuBeshter B, Warshal DP, Angel C, Dvoretsky PM, Lin JY, Raubertas RF. Endometrial carcinoma: the relevance of cervical cytology. Obstet Gynecol. 1991;77(3):458–62.

17. Roelofsen T, Geels YP, Pijnenborg JM, van Ham MA, Zomer SF, van Tilburg JM, et al. Cervical cytology in serous and endometrioid endometrial cancer. Int J Gynecol Pathol. 2013;32(4):390–8.

18. Brown AK, Gillis S, Deuel C, Angel C, Glantz C, Dubeshter B. Abnormal cervical cytology: a risk factor for endometrial cancer recurrence. Int J Gynecol Cancer. 2005;15(3):517–22.

19. Diaz-Rosario LA, Kabawat SE. Performance of a fluid-based, thin-layer papanicolaou smear method in the clinical setting of an independent laboratory and an outpatient screening population in New England. Arch Pathol Lab Med. 1999;123(9):817–21.

20. Misdraji J, Vaidya A, Tambouret RH, Duska L, Bell DA. Psammoma bodies in cervicovaginal cytology specimens: a clinicopathological analysis of 31 cases. Gynecol Oncol. 2006; 103(1):238–46.

21. Costa MJ, Kenny MB, Naib ZM. Cervicovaginal cytology in uterine adenocarcinoma and adenosquamous carcinoma. Comparison of cytologic and histologic findings. Acta Cytol. 1991;35(1):127–34.

22. Snyder MJ, Robboy SJ, Vollmer RT, Dodd LG. An abnormal cervicovaginal cytology smear in uterine carcinosarcoma is an adverse prognostic sign: analysis of 25 cases. Am J Clin Pathol. 2004;122(3):434–9.

23. Tambouret R, Pitman MB, Bell DA. Benign glandular cells in posthysterectomy vaginal smears. Acta Cytol. 1998; 42(6):1403–8.

# Chapter 7
# Cytology of Extracervical Adenocarcinoma

Except for the occasional adenocarcinoma of the endometrium, the appearance of extracervical adenocarcinoma in cervical cytology samples is rare. One large series reported 33 cases out of approximately 900,000 cervical cytology samples over a 22-year period for a rate of 0.004 % [1]. As was described in Chap. 6 for endometrial adenocarcinoma, extracervical adenocarcinoma may be directly sampled if the metastatic tumor has spread to the cervix or if the tumor cells have spontaneously detached from a location proximal to the cervix and shed down the fallopian tube and uterine corpus to be found as exfoliated cells in the cervical cytology sample. Adenocarcinoma is by far the most common variety of extracervical malignancy to present in cervical cytology [2]. A number of series detailing the surgical pathology findings of metastatic disease to the cervix have been published but rarely is adenocarcinoma in cervical cytology the trigger for clinical work-up [3–6]. This may be due to clinical practice variation as some institutions routinely obtain cervical cytology on all female cancer patients, even with known metastatic disease involving the cervix. Thus as reported in a recent Mexican series all 10 women with extracervical adenocarcinoma had cervical cytology with five smears positive for malignant cells [6]. Usually, patients having extracervical disease involving the cervix present with vaginal bleeding.

R.H. Tambouret and D.C. Wilbur, *Glandular Lesions of the Uterine Cervix*, Essentials in Cytopathology 19, DOI 10.1007/978-1-4939-1989-5_7, © Springer Science+Business Media New York 2015

Most often metastases to the cervix are identified at the time of the primary tumor diagnosis but cervical cytology can occasionally be the first manifestation of the primary cancer. In a few cases, the patients had no known malignancy making recognition of an extracervical primary important. The average age varies from 41 to 62 years, but a significant number of women in each series is younger than 40 years of age [3–6].

Primary tumors may arise from the genital tract or may be extragenital. The genital tumors most likely to be found in the cervix, in order of frequency are from the endometrium, ovary, fallopian tube, and primary peritoneal serous carcinoma. The extragenital organs most likely to give rise to metastatic adenocarcinoma to the cervix include tumors of the breast, stomach, and colon. Other less common sites include pancreas, gall bladder, appendix, and lung.

On cytology as well as surgical pathology, the morphology of metastatic adenocarcinoma in the cervix can be deceptively similar to a primary cervical adenocarcinoma due to predominant or exclusive mucosal involvement with morphologic resemblance to endocervical glandular epithelium [7–9]. However, most extracervical tumors exhibit features that suggest an origin from non-cervical sites, either by the tumor morphology or by the histologic pattern of involvement of the cervix.

# Cytomorphology of Metastatic Tumors

Although certain types of adenocarcinomas may have cytologic characteristics which suggest the organ of origin, many of the more common metastatic adenocarcinomas found in cervical cytology have overlapping features which do not permit on morphology alone to distinguish one tumor from another. The more common metastatic sites include tumors arising from the ovary, colon, stomach, and breast [3, 4, 6]. Cytologic features common to adenocarcinomas include the smear background which may or may not contain evidence of necrosis [10]. The tumor cells are often present as a combination of single cells and three-dimensional groups with

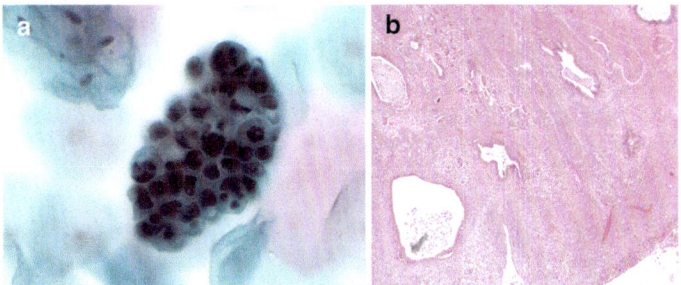

Fig. 7.1 Post-hysterectomy vaginal smear with a cluster of malignant glandular cells with prominent nucleoli and delicate cytoplasm consistent with recurrent endocervical adenocarcinoma (**a**); high power, SurePath, Papanicolaou stain; the subsequent biopsy showed the invasive recurrent adenocarcinoma (**b**); low power, hematoxylin and eosin

large hyperchromatic nuclei rimmed by irregular, thickened nuclear membranes. Nucleoli are usually strikingly prominent. The cytoplasm is usually delicate and variably vacuolated (Fig. 7.1). The number of tumor cells present may be few to many, depending on the site of gynecologic tract involvement. For tumors involving the lower tract, where direct sampling or many exfoliated cells occur, the numbers may be high. But in tumors originating in the upper gynecologic tract, where only a few cells may travel though the fallopian tubes and uterine corpus, the numbers of tumor cells seen in cervical specimens can be very low. A paucity of abnormal glandular cells is one reason that a definitive diagnosis of extragenital adenocarcinoma may not be made on a cervical cytology sample [1].

Certain morphologic clues may help determine the origin of the metastatic adenocarcinoma. The papillae of serous carcinoma of the endometrium, ovary, fallopian tube, and peritoneum most often present in cervical cytology as three-dimensional clusters of glandular cells due to exfoliation [11] (Fig. 7.2). The cells have abundant, clear (soap bubble-like) cytoplasm and hyperchromatic, eccentrically placed large nuclei with prominent nucleoli [1, 12] (Fig. 7.3). Less common

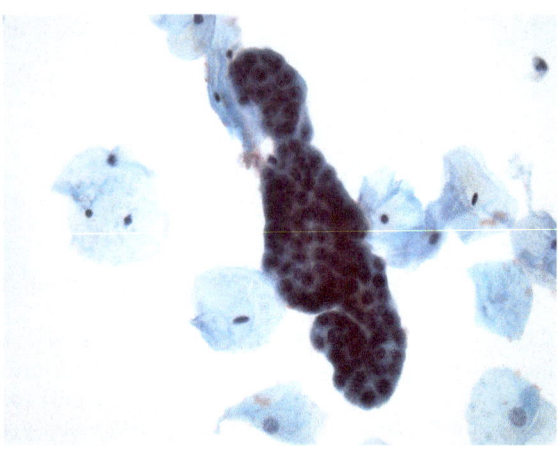

FIG. 7.2 Serous carcinoma present as a frond-like cluster; high power, SurePath, Papanicolaou stain

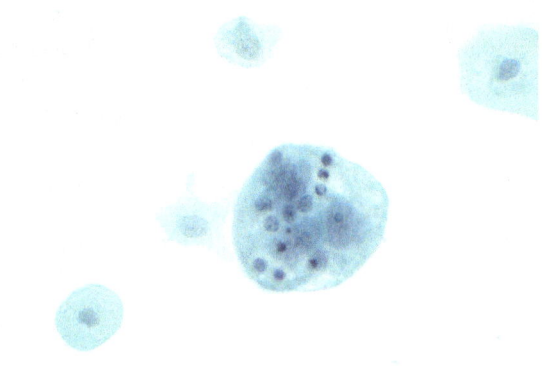

FIG. 7.3 A soap bubble appearance of serous carcinoma caused by the voluminous intracytoplasmic vacuoles; high power, SurePath, Papanicolaou stain

are frond-like papillary tissue fragments often associated with psammoma bodies (Fig. 7.4). Most often no evidence of tumor diathesis (necrosis or lysed blood) is present but some cases can show evidence of background necrosis or granular

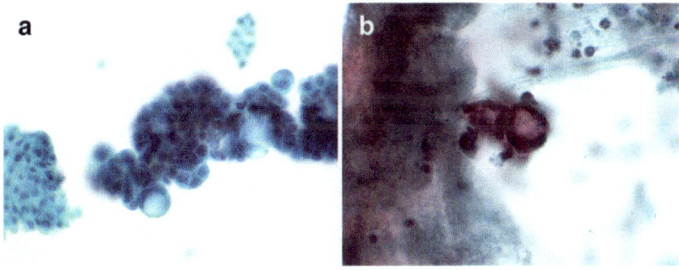

FIG. 7.4 Serous carcinoma with focally vacuolated cytoplasm present as an elongate group of cells (**a**); a psammoma body is surrounded by compressed tumor cells (**b**); both images high power, SurePath, Papanicolaou stain

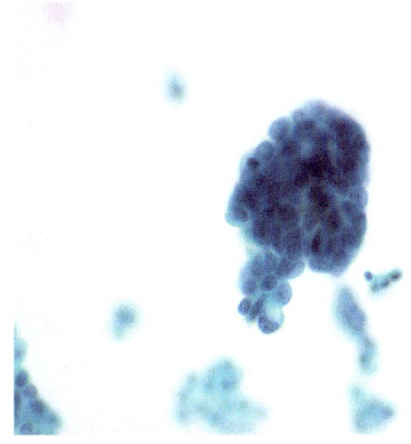

FIG. 7.5 Low grade serous borderline tumor cells with small nuclei tightly compressed into a compact three-dimensional cluster; high power, SurePath, Papanicolaou stain

debris [1]. Serous borderline tumors will resemble serous carcinoma in their three-dimensional cell arrangement but the nuclei are more often uniform with little of the pleomorphism of size and shape noted in fully malignant serous neoplasms [13] (Fig. 7.5).

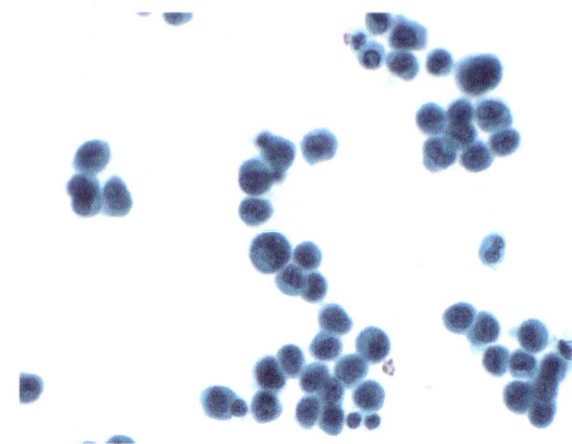

FIG. 7.6 Single cells of gastric carcinoma with variable high nuclear to cytoplasmic ratios, plus a few cells with prominent single intracytoplasmic vacuoles; high power, SurePath, Papanicolaou stain

Signet ring adenocarcinoma, usually from a gastric primary tumor, is morphologically identified in cytology samples by the presence of single malignant epithelial cells with a large intracytoplasmic vacuole that compresses the nucleus to edge of the cell [10] (Fig. 7.6).

Lobular carcinoma of the breast will usually produce single and small groups of malignant epithelial cells often with an eccentrically positioned round hyperchromatic nucleus containing a distinct nucleolus, giving the cell a somewhat plasmacytoid appearance [14] (Fig. 7.7). The cells of lobular carcinoma tend to be small with a high nuclear to cytoplasmic ratio, a nucleus larger than the nucleus of an intermediate squamous cell and the cytoplasm may contain a solitary vacuole pushing the nucleus to the periphery of the cell [15, 16] (Fig. 7.8). If the majority of tumor cells are vacuolated a designation of signet ring carcinoma may be warranted [17].

Metastatic adenocarcinoma from the colon will usually produce strips of malignant glandular cells having cigar-shaped hyperchromatic nuclei in a staggered array (Fig. 7.9). Colonic tumors are notorious for being associated with

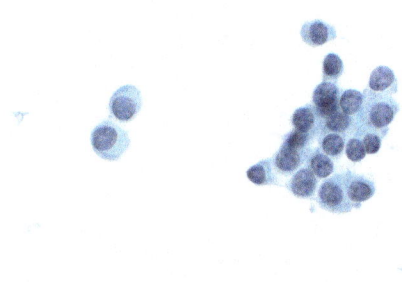

FIG. 7.7  Lobular carcinoma of the breast appears as small uniform cells with round uniform nuclei which are sometimes eccentrically positioned giving the cell a plasmacytoid appearance; high power, SurePath, Papanicolaou stain

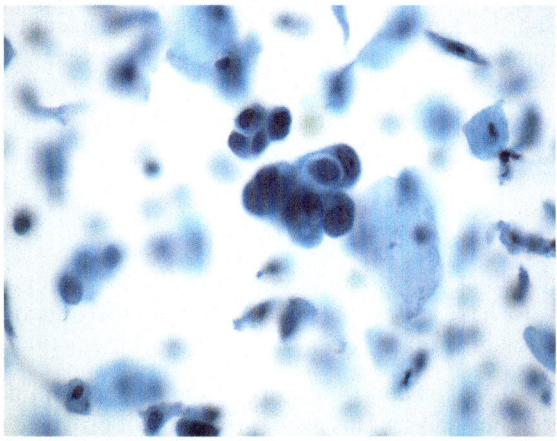

FIG. 7.8  Cells of lobular carcinoma may have solitary intracytoplasmic vacuoles as seen in this small cluster of malignant cells; high power, SurePath, Papanicolaou stain

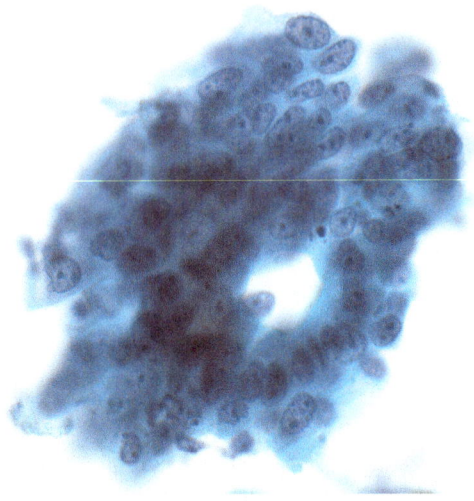

Fig. 7.9 The cells of metastatic colonic adenocarcinoma show glandular formation with round to cigar shaped nuclei; high power, SurePath, Papanicolaou stain

abundant background necrosis. In the case of rectal adenocarcinomas, direct tumor extension via recto-vaginal fistulas result in fecal material (vegetable or meat cells) in the cervical cytology sample in addition to tumor cells (Fig. 7.10).

## Work-up

If a glandular lesion identified on cervical cytology is suspected to have arisen outside of the endometrium, several steps should be taken.

*History of malignancy*: A history of malignancy will help to focus on the analysis. This history is often not provided to the pathologist the specimen requisition and should therefore be sought from the patient record. The abnormal cells in the cervical cytology sample can be compared to cytology or histology of any samples of the suspected primary tumor.

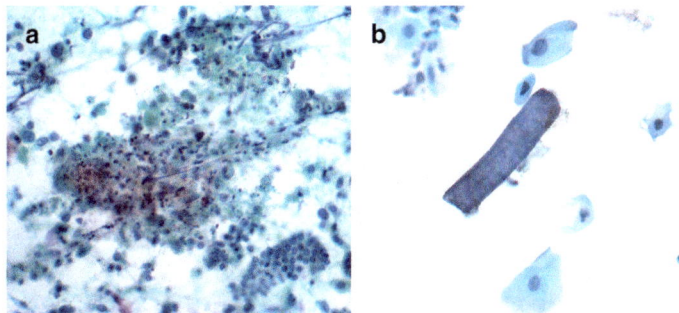

Fig. 7.10 If rectal carcinoma invades the cervix, a fistula may form. On cervical cytology abundant necrotic tissue may be identified (**a**) as well as vegetable material such as the rectangular shaped structure in this image (**b**); both images high power, SurePath, Papanicolaou stain

*High risk HPV testing*: Because most primary adenocarcinomas of the endocervix are positive for high risk HPV, testing of the residual material in the cytology sample is a practical step to help narrow the choices and is especially important in metastatic carcinomas that mimic primary cervical adenocarcinoma, such as endometrial or colonic tumors [7].

*Cell block preparation*: Liquid-based cytology samples afford the opportunity to utilize the residual sample for the preparation of a cell block (see Chap. 2) (Fig. 7.11) Cell blocks allow histologic evaluation of the abnormal cells, particularly architectural assessment of groups, and hence comparison to prior tumors are removed from the patient. Special stains, such as mucicarmine or immunohistochemical and in situ hybridization studies can be performed. For example, testing for high risk HPV can be done by in situ hybridization in order to see if any positive results obtained are actually from the tumor cells in question [7].

*Immunohistochemical stains*: If a cell block is prepared and the number of abnormal cells is sufficient, immunohistochemical stains may be very helpful. Because the majority of cervical adenocarcinomas are associated with high risk HPV,

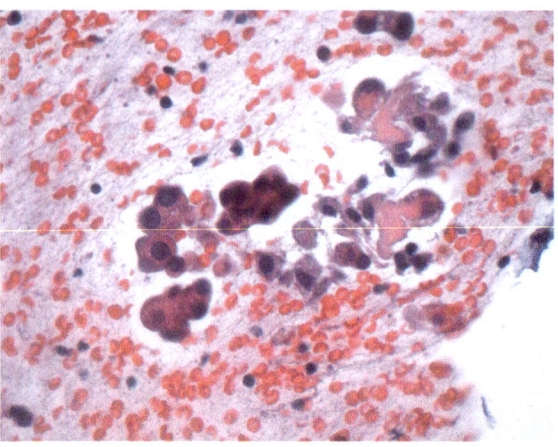

FIG. 7.11  A cell block was made from the SurePath cervical cytology vial (Fig. 7.2); hematoxylin-eosin, high power section showing small clusters of serous carcinoma; the multiple histologic sections which can be obtained from the cell block are useful for special stains

mainly HPV 16 and 18, immunohistochemical staining or in situ hybridization may be performed [18–20]. However, most of the less common types of endocervical adenocarcinoma, such as minimal deviation, gastric-type, intestinal-type, mesonephric and clear cell are not related to HPV infection [21]. p16 may be used as a surrogate marker for the presence of HPV but p16 is also overexpressed in certain extracervical tumors such as serous carcinoma of the uterine corpus [22]. Testing for estrogen and progesterone receptors are usually part of a panel to differentiate endocervical (negative) from endometrial (positive) adenocarcinoma [19]. Studies have supported the use of CEA and vimentin in addition to other markers [23, 24] to distinguish endocervical adenocarcinoma from adenocarcinoma originating from the endometrium. However, the use of CEA and vimentin has not been found to be helpful in all instances as the staining pattern is not uniform in all variants arising for a given site of origin [25, 26]. Examples of useful antibodies include TTF-1 and Napsin A for lung adenocarcinoma [27], cytokeratin (CK) 7, CK20, and

TABLE 7.1 Adenocarcinoma arising in different organs and corresponding immunohistochemical stains useful on cervical cytology cell blocks

| Primary site of ACA | Positive in majority of cases |
| --- | --- |
| Endocervix | HPV, p16 |
| Endometrium | ER, PR |
| Lung | TTF-1, Napsin-A |
| Lower GI | CK20, CDX2 |
| Upper GI | CDX2, CK17, CK7, MUC1, MUC2 |
| Breast | GATA3, ER |

*HPV* human papillomavirus, *ER* estrogen receptor, *PR* progesterone receptor, *TTF-1* thyroid transcription factor-1, *CK* cytokeratin, *MUC* mucin

CDX2 for lower gastrointestinal adenocarcinoma [28–30], CDX2, CK17, MUC1, and MUC2 for adenocarcinomas of the upper gastrointestinal tract [31, 32] and GATA3 and estrogen receptor for breast tumors [33]. The immunohistochemical panels are summarized in Table 7.1.

A particular problem occurs in determination of the site of origin of mucinous adenocarcinoma. These tumors arise from a variety of organs and yet have a remarkably similar morphology. They are composed of either glands lined by mucin-producing cells with abundant extracellular mucin comprising more than 50 % of the tumor mass or mucin-containing signet ring cells. A recent review of immunohistochemistry to distinguish between primary and metastatic ovarian mucinous neoplasms found a significant degree of overlap between the intestinal-type of ovarian tumors and tumors of the upper gastrointestinal tract when a panel of nine markers was used (CK7, CK20, CEA, CA19.9, CDX2, CA125, ER, DPC4, and p16) [34]. However, another immunohistochemical algorithm using a panel of ten markers (CK7, CK20, CDX-2, β-catenin, MUC-1, MUC-2, MUC-6, ER, WT-1, and PAX-8) has been tested and found useful in determining the primary site; the profiles are summarized in Table 7.2 [35].

*Molecular profiling*: Identification of a primary tumor site by molecular tumor profiling has been studied as a complement or alternative to immunohistochemical staining [36–38]. The limitation in cell block samples will probably be the amount of tumor cells present.

TABLE 7.2 Suggested immunohistochemical panels for diverse mucinous adenocarcinomas [33, 35, 40]

| Organ of origin | Positive results | Negative results |
| --- | --- | --- |
| Cervix | CK7, MUC1, MUC6, ER | CK20, CDX2, nuclear β-catenin |
| Endometrium | CK7, MUC1, PAX8, ER | CK20, CDX2, nuclear β-catenin |
| Ovary | PAX8, CK7, CDX2 (heterogeneous), ER (stromal) | MUC6, WT1, nuclear β-catenin |
| Colon | CK7 (CK7 may be positive (40 % focal, 10 % extensive) or negative (50 %) in colorectal adenocarcinoma), CK20, CDX2 (homogeneous), MUC2, nuclear β-catenin | CK7, MUC1, MUC6 |
| Rectum/anus | CK7 (positive in anal gland carcinoma), CK20 (negative in anal gland carcinoma), CDX2 (homogeneous), MUC2, nuclear β-catenin | MUC1, MUC6 |
| Appendix | CK7, CK20, CDX2 (heterogeneous), MUC2 | MUC1, MUC6, nuclear β-catenin |
| Upper GI | CK7, CK20, CDX2 (heterogeneous), MUC2, MUC6 | ER, WT1, PAX8 |
| Bladder | CK7, CK20, CDX2 (heterogeneous), MUC2 | MUC1, MUC6, nuclear β-catenin, GATA3 |
| Breast | CK7, MUC1, MUC2, MUC6, ER, WT1, GATA3 | CK20, CDX2, nuclear β-catenin |
| Lung | | |

*CK* cytokeratin, *MUC* mucin, *ER* estrogen receptor

# The Future

While morphologic evidence of extracervical adenocarcinoma may be a rare event in cervical cytology specimens, researchers are currently exploring the possibility that cervical cytology samples can be a source of tumor DNA to screen for ovarian and endometrial cancers [39]. Early success has been reported when sophisticated molecular techniques are used to detect oncogenic DNA mutations as specific clonal markers of the presence of ovarian and endometrial cancer cells.

# References

1. Gupta D, Balsara G. Extrauterine malignancies. Role of Pap smears in diagnosis and management. Acta Cytol. 1999;43(5):806–13.
2. Ng AB, Reagan JW, Hawliczek S, Wentz BW. Significance of endometrial cells in the detection of endometrial carcinoma and its precursors. Acta Cytol. 1974;18(5):356–61.
3. Mazur MT, Hsueh S, Gersell DJ. Metastases to the female genital tract. Analysis of 325 cases. Cancer. 1984;53(9):1978–84.
4. Lemoine NR, Hall PA. Epithelial tumors metastatic to the uterine cervix. A study of 33 cases and review of the literature. Cancer. 1986;57(10):2002–5.
5. Mulvany N, Ostor A. Microinvasive adenocarcinoma of the cervix: a cytohistopathologic study of 40 cases. Diagn Cytopathol. 1997;16(5):430–6.
6. Perez-Montiel D, Serrano-Olvera A, Salazar LC, Cetina-Perez L, Candelaria M, Coronel J, et al. Adenocarcinoma metastatic to the uterine cervix: a case series. J Obstet Gynaecol Res. 2012; 38(3):541–9.
7. McCluggage WG, Hurrell DP, Kennedy K. Metastatic carcinomas in the cervix mimicking primary cervical adenocarcinoma and adenocarcinoma in situ: report of a series of cases. Am J Surg Pathol. 2010;34(5):735–41.
8. Malpica A, Deavers MT. Ovarian low-grade serous carcinoma involving the cervix mimicking a cervical primary. Int J Gynecol Pathol. 2011;30(6):613–9.
9. Matsushita H, Fukase M, Takayanagi T, Ikarashi H. Metastatic gastric cancer mimicking an advanced cervical cancer: a case report. Eur J Gynaecol Oncol. 2011;32(2):199–200.
10. Kashimura M, Kashimura Y, Matsuyama T, Tsukamoto N, Sugimori H, Taki I. Adenocarcinoma of the uterine cervix metastatic from primary stomach cancer. Cytologic findings in six cases. Acta Cytol. 1983;27(1):54–8.

11. Wang H, Chen PC. Primary serous peritoneal carcinoma presenting first on a routine papanicolaou smear: a case report. Acta Cytol. 2010;54(4):623–6.

12. Wilbur DC, Henry MR, editors. College of American Pathologists practical guide to gynecologic cytopathology: morphology, management, and molecular methods. Northfield: College of American Pathologists; 2008.

13. Tepeoglu M, Ozen O, Ayhan A. Ovarian serous borderline tumor detected by conventional papanicolaou smear: a case report. Acta Cytol. 2013;57(1):96–9.

14. McKee GT. Cytopathology of the Breast. New York: Oxford University Press; 2002.

15. Rau AR, Saldanha P, Raghuveer CV. Metastatic lobular mammary carcinoma diagnosed in cervicovaginal smears: a case report. Diagn Cytopathol. 2003;29(5):300–2.

16. Haji BE, Kapila K, Francis IM, Temmim L, Ahmed MS. Cytomorphological features of metastatic mammary lobular carcinoma in cervicovaginal smears: report of a case and review of literature. Cytopathology. 2005;16(1):42–8.

17. Pambuccian SE, Bachowski GJ, Twiggs LB. Signet ring cell lobular carcinoma of the breast presenting in a cervicovaginal smear. A case report. Acta Cytol. 2000;44(5):824–30.

18. Pirog EC, Kleter B, Olgac S, Bobkiewicz P, Lindeman J, Quint WG, et al. Prevalence of human papillomavirus DNA in different histological subtypes of cervical adenocarcinoma. Am J Pathol. 2000;157(4):1055–62.

19. Yemelyanova A, Vang R, Seidman JD, Gravitt PE, Ronnett BM. Endocervical adenocarcinomas with prominent endometrial or endomyometrial involvement simulating primary endometrial carcinomas: utility of HPV DNA detection and immunohistochemical expression of p16 and hormone receptors to confirm the cervical origin of the corpus tumor. Am J Surg Pathol. 2009;33(6):914–24.

20. Kong CS, Beck AH, Longacre TA. A panel of 3 markers including p16, ProExC, or HPV ISH is optimal for distinguishing between primary endometrial and endocervical adenocarcinomas. Am J Surg Pathol. 2010;34(7):915–26.

21. Park KJ, Kiyokawa T, Soslow RA, Lamb CA, Oliva E, Zivanovic O, et al. Unusual endocervical adenocarcinomas: an immunohistochemical analysis with molecular detection of human papillomavirus. Am J Surg Pathol. 2011;35(5):633–46.

22. Yemelyanova A, Ji H, Shih Ie M, Wang TL, Wu LS, Ronnett BM. Utility of p16 expression for distinction of uterine serous

carcinomas from endometrial endometrioid and endocervical adenocarcinomas: immunohistochemical analysis of 201 cases. Am J Surg Pathol. 2009;33(10):1504–14.

23. McCluggage WG, Sumathi VP, McBride HA, Patterson A. A panel of immunohistochemical stains, including carcinoembryonic antigen, vimentin, and estrogen receptor, aids the distinction between primary endometrial and endocervical adenocarcinomas. Int J Gynecol Pathol. 2002;21(1):11–5.

24. Zaino RJ. Symposium part I: adenocarcinoma in situ, glandular dysplasia, and early invasive adenocarcinoma of the uterine cervix. Int J Gynecol Pathol. 2002;21(4):314–26.

25. Kamoi S, AlJuboury MI, Akin MR, Silverberg SG. Immunohistochemical staining in the distinction between primary endometrial and endocervical adenocarcinomas: another viewpoint. Int J Gynecol Pathol. 2002;21(3):217–23.

26. Kurman RJ, Ellenson LH, Ronnett BM. Blausteins's pathology of the female genital tract. 6th ed. New York: Springer; 2011.

27. Fatima N, Cohen C, Lawson D, Siddiqui MT. TTF-1 and Napsin A double stain: a useful marker for diagnosing lung adenocarcinoma on fine-needle aspiration cell blocks. Cancer Cytopathol. 2011;119(2):127–33.

28. Chu P, Wu E, Weiss LM. Cytokeratin 7 and cytokeratin 20 expression in epithelial neoplasms: a survey of 435 cases. Mod Pathol. 2000;13(9):962–72.

29. Werling RW, Yaziji H, Bacchi CE, Gown AM. CDX2, a highly sensitive and specific marker of adenocarcinomas of intestinal origin: an immunohistochemical survey of 476 primary and metastatic carcinomas. Am J Surg Pathol. 2003;27(3):303–10.

30. Vang R, Gown AM, Wu LS, Barry TS, Wheeler DT, Yemelyanova A, et al. Immunohistochemical expression of CDX2 in primary ovarian mucinous tumors and metastatic mucinous carcinomas involving the ovary: comparison with CK20 and correlation with coordinate expression of CK7. Mod Pathol. 2006;19(11):1421–8.

31. Chu PG, Schwarz RE, Lau SK, Yen Y, Weiss LM. Immunohistochemical staining in the diagnosis of pancreatobiliary and ampulla of Vater adenocarcinoma: application of CDX2, CK17, MUC1, and MUC2. Am J Surg Pathol. 2005;29(3):359–67.

32. Yang HS, Tamayo R, Almonte M, Horten B, DaSilva M, Gangi M, et al. Clinical significance of MUC1, MUC2 and CK17 expression patterns for diagnosis of pancreatobiliary arcinoma. Biotech Histochem. 2012;87(2):126–32.

33. Ordonez NG. Value of GATA3 immunostaining in tumor diagnosis: a review. Adv Anat Pathol. 2013;20(5):352–60.

34. McCluggage WG. Immunohistochemistry in the distinction between primary and metastatic ovarian mucinous neoplasms. J Clin Pathol. 2012;65(7):596–600.
35. Chu PG, Chung L, Weiss LM, Lau SK. Determining the site of origin of mucinous adenocarcinoma: an immunohistochemical study of 175 cases. Am J Surg Pathol. 2011;35(12):1830–6.
36. Greco FA, Lennington WJ, Spigel DR, Hainsworth JD. Molecular profiling diagnosis in unknown primary cancer: accuracy and ability to complement standard pathology. J Natl Cancer Inst. 2013;105(11):782–90.
37. Greco FA, Oien K, Erlander M, Osborne R, Varadhachary G, Bridgewater J, et al. Cancer of unknown primary: progress in the search for improved and rapid diagnosis leading toward superior patient outcomes. Ann Oncol. 2012;23(2):298–304.
38. Handorf CR, Kulkarni A, Grenert JP, Weiss LM, Rogers WM, Kim OS, et al. A multicenter study directly comparing the diagnostic accuracy of gene expression profiling and immunohistochemistry for primary site identification in metastatic tumors. Am J Surg Pathol. 2013;37(7):1067–75.
39. Kinde I, Bettegowda C, Wang Y, Wu J, Agrawal N, Shih IM, et al. Evaluation of DNA from the Papanicolaou test to detect ovarian and endometrial cancers. Sci Transl Med. 2013;5(167):167ra4.
40. Ordonez NG. Value of PAX 8 immunostaining in tumor diagnosis: a review and update. Adv Anat Pathol. 2012;19(3):140–51.

# Chapter 8

## Management of Glandular Lesions Identified on Cervical Cytology and Histology with Suggestions for Continuous Quality Improvement in the Cytology Laboratory

### Rational for Management Guidelines

Following the publication of the revised Bethesda System terminology for reporting cervical cytology results and the revised guidelines for cervical cancer screening in 2001, the American Society for Colposcopy and Cervical Pathology (ASCCP) convened a consensus forum for the development of evidence-based guidelines for management of women with abnormal cervical cytology, cervical intraepithelial neoplasia (CIN), and adenocarcinoma in situ (AIS). The first management guidelines were published in 2002 with revisions published in 2007 and most recently in 2013 [1].

The following describes the management guidelines for cytology interpretations of glandular lesions identified in cervical cytology samples.

R.H. Tambouret and D.C. Wilbur, *Glandular Lesions of the Uterine Cervix*, Essentials in Cytopathology 19, DOI 10.1007/978-1-4939-1989-5_8,

The interpretation of atypical glandular cells (AGC) on cervical cytology is not common and the cytologic criteria have been found to be poorly reproducible. The spectrum of underlying pathology leading to the interpretation of AGC can vary from benign reparative processes, metaplasia, endocervical polyps, and changes secondary to intrauterine devices to adenocarcinomas of the cervix, endometrium, fallopian tubes, ovaries, and more distant sites as detailed in earlier chapters of this monograph. The AGC interpretation can be qualified by "favor neoplasia" which is associated with a higher risk of serious pathology. Although the cytologic criteria for the recognition of AIS have been refined over the years, an interpretation of AIS is uncommonly made on cytology samples in comparison to the more common AGC categorization. The risk of neoplasia or preneoplasia following the interpretation of AGC has been reported to be 29 % [2]. The most common underlying pathology in patients with AGC cytology is squamous dysplasia including LSIL. Squamous dysplasia is found in association with AIS in about 50 % of women diagnosed with AIS. The risk of pathology is increased when concurrent ASC-US is present. The risk of CIN2+ is increased in younger women while the risk of underlying carcinoma is higher in older women [3]. Except for young women with a genetic predisposition, the risk of endometrial adenocarcinoma is especially high in older women. A large study from California found the risk of CIN3+ was 9 % following a cytologic interpretation of AGC and the risk of carcinoma was 3 % [4]. Although endocervical adenocarcinoma and AIS are associated with HPV in the majority of cases, adenocarcinoma or hyperplasia of the endometrium is not, so testing for HPV will not help triage women who need additional investigation. But a negative HPV test can suggest an endometrial origin rather than endocervical lesion [5]. Other potential cytologic clues of underlying endometrial disease are the presence of benign-appearing endometrial glandular cells or stromal cells in women over 40 years of age, especially those who have exited their reproductive years.

# Management Guidelines for the Cytologic Interpretation of "Atypical Glandular Cells" or "Adenocarcinoma In Situ"

Management of all subcategories of AGC should always prompt colposcopy with endocervical sampling (Table 8.1). HPV testing is not recommended because colposcopy is advised regardless of HPV status; however, if an HPV test is obtained it can be used in the downstream management of the patient following the initial work-up. Likewise, repeat cervical cytology should not be considered as the primary follow-up of these diagnoses. In women aged 35 and older or in younger women with risk factors for endometrial adenocarcinoma, sampling of the endometrium should be performed along with colposcopy and sampling of the endocervical canal. Risk factors for endometrial adenocarcinoma in younger women include abnormal vaginal bleeding and chronic anovulation.

In the setting of atypical endometrial cells, sampling of the endometrium and endocervical canal should be performed but colposcopy may be deferred until the results of endometrial and endocervical samples are finalized. If no pathology is identified, colposcopy should then be performed, because of the possibility of endometrioid neoplastic lesions of the cervix as have been previously described.

In the setting of AGC—not otherwise specified, in which there is no evidence of CIN2+ identified on biopsy, the guidelines recommend follow-up co-testing with cytology

TABLE 8.1 Initial patient work-up following identification of AGC on cytology

1. All subcategories of AGC except atypical endometrial cells
   - Colposcopy with endocervical sampling
   - Add endometrial sampling if patient >35 years or is at risk for endometrial neoplasia
2. Atypical endometrial cells
   - Endometrial and endocervical sampling
   - Colposcopy only if no endometrial pathology is identified following above samples

*AGC* atypical glandular cells

Table 8.2  Subsequent patient management of AGC

1. Initial cytology was AGC, not otherwise specified
   – No HSIL, AIS, or carcinoma identified
   – Cotest for HPV and cytology at 12 and 24 months
     – If 12 and 24 month tests negative, cotest 3 years later
     – If any abnormalities are identified, patient undergoes colposcopy
2. Initial cytology was AGC favor neoplasia or AIS
   – If no invasive disease identified on colposcopic biopsies, proceed to diagnostic excisional procedure with evaluation of tissue margins

*AGC* atypical glandular cells, *HSIL* high grade squamous intraepithelial lesion, *AIS* adenocarcinoma in situ, *HPV* human papillomavirus

Table 8.3  Management of patients diagnosed with AIS on diagnostic excisional procedure

1. Hysterectomy—preferred if childbearing is completed
2. Fertility sparing conservative management
   – If margins negative, proceed with long-term follow-up
   – If margins are involved or ECC is positive
     – Reexcision is the recommended follow-up
     – Reevaluation with HPV and cytology co-testing, colposcopy, and endocervical sampling at 6 months is acceptable

*AIS* adenocarcinoma in situ, *ECC* endocervical curettage, *HPV* human papillomavirus

and HPV at 12 and 24 months (Table 8.2). If the additional tests are negative, the patient should return for repeat co-testing in 3 years. If abnormal results are found on any of the tests, the patient should be evaluated with colposcopy.

If the initial work-up of atypical endocervical cells, atypical endometrial cells or AGCs—not otherwise specified, is diagnostic for CIN2+ without evidence of glandular neoplasia, the management should follow the 2012 guidelines for the lesion that is found.

If the initial colposcopic work-up for women with AGC—favor neoplasia or endocervical AIS on cytology reveals no evidence of invasive tumor, a diagnostic excisional procedure which provides sufficient tissue to evaluate margins is recommended. Also, endocervical sampling after the excision should be performed. Clinical management of patients diagnosed with AIS on biopsy depends on the desire for preserved fertility (Table 8.3).

# Management Guidelines for the Cytologic Interpretation of "Atypical Glandular Cells" or "Adenocarcinoma In Situ" in Special Populations: Pregnant Women and Women Aged 21–24 Years

In pregnant women with AGC on cytology, the initial evaluation should consist of colposcopy but endocervical and endometrial sampling should not be performed.

In women aged 21–24 years with AGC on cytology, the management should be the same as for women over the age of 24 years.

## Management of Benign Glandular Cells

The finding of benign endometrial glandular or stromal cells in asymptomatic premenopausal women does not require further evaluation; however, in postmenopausal women assessment of the endometrium is recommended. For women over 40 who have benign-appearing endometrial cells in their cervical cytology specimens, TBS recommends reporting these as such. Some laboratories modify this recommendation, only reporting such findings if there is either no menstrual history available or if the cells appear out of phase (in the second half of the menstrual cycle). If any of these circumstances is present, it is then up to the clinician to decide, based on the overall history and physical findings, if further tests are warranted.

In women who have undergone a hysterectomy and in whom benign glandular cells are identified on cytology, no additional evaluation is recommended.

Management of women with cytologic AIS is less straightforward than management of women with high grade squamous lesions. AIS tends to be more often hidden from view in the endocervical canal, such that the colposcopic changes of AIS are minimal. Although AIS may rarely be multifocal within the endocervical canal with areas of intervening normal endocervical epithelium, these lesions are most commonly continuous and may involve multiple quadrants [6, 7]. Determination of extent of disease is difficult which complicates the surgical calculation of the depth of excision. An excisional procedure (loop excision or knife cone biopsy) is necessary to exclude the presence of invasion. The first step in management is performance of colposcopy with excisional biopsy of any visible lesions and sampling of the endocervical canal by curettage in order to obtain histologic confirmation of AIS. Once the histologic diagnosis is established additional management depends on the reproductive history. For women who want to maintain fertility, more conservative management is acceptable. If the margins of the excisional biopsy or the endocervical sampling contain squamous intraepithelial lesion or AIS, reexcision is preferred. The woman should undergo reevaluation at 6 months with colposcopy, cytology, and HPV testing.

# Continuous Quality Improvement in the Cytology Laboratory

In conclusion, several basic tenets of endocervical glandular abnormality management should be highlighted. First, glandular lesions of the cervix are rare and cytologic interpretations of AGC and higher should be made only rarely. CAP and other literature data suggest that the prevalence of AGC interpretations in the laboratory should be less than 1 % and often much lower, with the CAP reporting laboratory mean being 0.3 %. Close monitoring of the prevalence of this interpretation in the laboratory, with investigation if the number of case exceeds this threshold, is very important in a quality management program. The pathologist is advised to seek additional clinical history any time an interpretation of AGC or more severe glandular lesion (AGC+) is entertained. Often history not initially available emerges which can be very helpful in the evaluation of the specimen. The most common additional historical information is the presence of an IUD, an endocervical polyp, or the presence of prior cervical disease, particularly of squamous origin with a prior cone procedure. Follow-up and cytology–histology correlation are also important in the quality management of glandular cervical lesions. This process allows for the development of greater experience and feedback on prior cytologically difficult cases and allows for the honing of criteria and their application. Adherence to these principles in the rare cases of AGC+seen on Pap tests can lead to overall improvements in accuracy of interpretation in this most challenging area of cervical cytology.

# References

1. Massad LS, Einstein MH, Huh WK, Katki HA, Kinney WK, Schiffman M, et al. 2012 updated consensus guidelines for the management of abnormal cervical cancer screening tests and cancer precursors. J Low Genit Tract Dis. 2013;17(5 Suppl 1):S1–27.
2. Schnatz PF, Guile M, O'Sullivan DM, Sorosky JI. Clinical significance of atypical glandular cells on cervical cytology. Obstet Gynecol. 2006;107(3):701–8.
3. Zhao C, Austin RM, Pan J, Barr N, Martin SE, Raza A, et al. Clinical significance of atypical glandular cells in conventional pap smears in a large, high-risk U.S. west coast minority population. Acta Cytol. 2009;53(2):153–9.
4. Katki HA, Schiffman M, Castle PE, Fetterman B, Poitras NE, Lorey T, et al. Five-year risks of CIN 3+ and cervical cancer among women with HPV-positive and HPV-negative high-grade Pap results. J Low Genit Tract Dis. 2013;17(5 Suppl 1):S50–5.
5. Castle PE, Fetterman B, Poitras N, Lorey T, Shaber R, Kinney W. Relationship of atypical glandular cell cytology, age, and human papillomavirus detection to cervical and endometrial cancer risks. Obstet Gynecol. 2010;115(2 Pt 1):243–8.
6. Ostor AG, Duncan A, Quinn M, Rome R. Adenocarcinoma in situ of the uterine cervix: an experience with 100 cases. Gynecol Oncol. 2000;79(2):207–10.
7. Zaino RJ. Symposium part I: adenocarcinoma in situ, glandular dysplasia, and early invasive adenocarcinoma of the uterine cervix. Int J Gynecol Pathol. 2002;21(4):314–26.

**ERRATUM**

# Glandular Lesions of the Uterine Cervix
## Cytopathology with Histologic Correlates

**Rosemary H. Tambouret and David C. Wilbur**

R.H. Tambouret and D.C. Wilbur, *Glandular Lesions of the Uterine Cervix*, Essentials in Cytopathology 19, DOI 10.1007/978-1-4939-1989-5, © Springer Science+Business Media New York 2015

**DOI 10.1007/978-1-4939-1989-5_9**

The authors for Foreword have been revised. The following revisions were made:
The authors "Rosemary H. Tambouret, Boston, MA, USA" and "David C. Wilbur, Boston, MA, USA" were replaced with "Robert H. Young, Boston, MA, USA" and "Robert E. Scully, Boston, MA, USA."

The online version of the original book can be found at
http://dx.doi.org/10.1007/978-1-4939-1989-5

# Index

R.H. Tambouret and D.C. Wilbur, *Glandular Lesions*
*of the Uterine Cervix*, Essentials in Cytopathology 19,
DOI 10.1007/978-1-4939-1989-5,
© Springer Science+Business Media New York 2015

The manufacturer's authorised representative in the EU is Springer
Nature Customer Service Centre GmbH, Europaplatz 3, 69115 Heidelberg,
Germany. If you have any concerns regarding our products, please
contact ProductSafety@springernature.com

Printed and bound by CPI Group (UK) Ltd, Croydon, CR0 4YY
23/04/2026
02095602-0002